Helping Children Become the Heroes of their Stories

Whether it's the anxiety of social isolation, the loss of routine or a breakdown in formal educational support, the COVID-19 pandemic has affected children in countless ways. Teachers, therapists and parents frequently find themselves ill-equipped to help children struggling with the difficult feelings that these situations, and others like them, give rise to.

This essential guide provides a therapeutic toolkit to enable children to tell their stories and to regain some control over their mental health and wellbeing. The toolkit introduces a therapeutic story template, alongside guided support and examples focusing on three therapeutic skill sets: active listening, reflection and handling questions. Designed for use with children both individually and in class groups, the storytelling toolkit will enable children to see themselves as the hero of their own story, and life, and to reinstate a sense of optimism and self-empowerment in the face of the pandemic challenge.

This resource provides a practical toolkit which can be used both inside and outside the classroom to help children to tell their lockdown stories. It will be valuable reading for teachers, SENCOs, therapists, mental health leads and parents.

Amanda Seyderhelm trains professionals and parents how to support grieving children and families through play and the creative arts. She is an experienced certified play therapist, having worked in private practice since 2016. Amanda was the creative arts lead of the Craft Station at Great Ormond Street Hospital for Children Charity for two years, and is now a partner agency with Barnardo's on loss and bereavement. She also consults for theatre in education groups in the community, www.helpingchildrensmileagain.com.

T0386624

Helping Children Become the Heroes of their Stories

A Practical Guide to Overcoming Adversity and Building Resilience in Every Setting

Amanda Seyderhelm

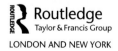

Routledge
Taylor & Francis Group

LONDON AND NEW YORK

Cover image: © Amanda Seyderhelm. Photo of spoon superheroes taken at the play therapy group at The Malcolm Sargent Primary School, Lincolnshire, formed to promote building peer relationships.

First published 2023
by Routledge
4 Park Square, Milton Park, Abingdon, Oxon OX14 4RN

and by Routledge
605 Third Avenue, New York, NY 10158

Routledge is an imprint of the Taylor & Francis Group, an informa business

British Library Cataloguing-in-Publication Data
A catalogue record for this book is available from the British Library

Library of Congress Cataloging-in-Publication Data
A catalog record has been requested for this book

ISBN: 978-1-032-02127-0 (hbk)
ISBN: 978-1-032-02124-9 (pbk)
ISBN: 978-1-003-18200-9 (ebk)

DOI: 10.4324/9781003182009

Typeset in Frutiger
by Deanta Global Publishing Services, Chennai, India

For the hero who lives within all of us.

Distorting Joe

Joe had a way of making things BIGGER
Than they actually were.
Blowing up buildings (on paper)
Shining a light on something small
And almost hidden.
Leaving out a word he didn't understand.
Saying what other people were desperate
To say.
Shrinking the truth, the obvious, painful.
Joe noticed, the more he **distorted**
The clearer
       Clearer

          Clearer
            Things became.
Joe started to wonder
         What **distorted** meant.
He asked his teacher,
His Dad
Random strangers,
Wilph, his friend from the park bench.
Ronnie at school,
And finally Thelma, who knew everything.
Distortion happens when you can't see the rest, she said.
The rest of what? asked Joe.
What's around the corner?
No.
The end of something?
No.
The start of something?
No.
Joe felt he could go on forever asking what 'the rest' meant.
I can understand why you might
Imagine all of those scenarios, said Thelma.

Around the corner is **fear**.
The end is <u>sad</u>.
The start is *anxiety*.
Joe looked even more confused.
His ears started to itch.
'The rest' is right here – inside. Beside. Alongside,
Wherever you choose to put 'the rest',
There it will be, said Thelma.
Joe had to sit down.
This was news to contemplate.
Why hadn't he read about 'the rest'?, he wondered,
Seen her on TV, on the news?
Why were people so quiet about 'the rest'?
His ears stopped itching.
People are so busy they forget 'the rest' is there, said Thelma,
So they see other things instead
And, the picture becomes …
DISTORTED! shouted Joe.
Thelma smiled.
My Dad is very busy, and tired, sighed Joe.
Maybe you can introduce him to 'the rest'?
What would that be like?, asked Thelma.
A whole new world, said Joe.

I wrote 'Distorting Joe' shortly after the UK, and the rest of the world, entered lockdown during the first wave of the COVID-19 pandemic. Millions of people died worldwide. We were shut inside our homes, isolated, socially distanced from one another. Our worlds shrank. Finding rest during this time was challenging. I created a new relationship with rest.

The story is published in *Healing Power of the Imagination Journal*, December 2021.

Quote from an 8-year-old boy

Me to a child: What is the one thing you wish you had had during this pandemic?
Child to me: A torch.

For most of us, the creative process resembles a quest. There is a gnawing sensation we carry deep within us that yearns for resolution.
(Maureen Murdock (1990), *The Heroine's Journey: Woman's Quest for Wholeness*.)

Contents

Foreword

Amanda Seyderhelm has over 15 years' experience of working as a certified creative play therapist for children between the ages of 4 and 12. She is someone we should listen to, and since I met Amanda over three years ago, her expertise and experiences have inspired me in my own practice.

After many years of helping and supporting hurting children, Amanda's tremendous drive continues to grow for wanting to make a positive difference to the lives of children who have suffered loss or change. Just about every child on planet Earth has undergone some change over the past 18 months during the global Covid-19 pandemic, and, sadly, many have also suffered loss. We are therefore talking about reaching children on a mass scale, far more perhaps than Amanda anticipated when she first set out on her journey as a play therapist some years ago.

We talk at length, Amanda and I, about the emotional landscape that exists in schools and homes. Despite our world being more IT savvy, apparently more connected and more sophisticated than ever before, the children we support and work with are struggling with fundamental human emotions and very obviously need help and specialist support. We are further saddened when we see an educator and/ or parent struggling to cope, and, in turn, unable to be there emotionally for the children in their care. Nobody wins. But who should help them? And how? What options are open to an adult whose job it is to educate and support a child if they don't have the training, expertise or resources? Already busy teachers, an increase in referrals to an already busy Child and Adult Mental Health Services (CAMHS) and educational-psychology teams and lack of funding for education are all factors that negate success for our children. Pile on the top the global pandemic and it's surely a recipe for running and taking cover for the most dedicated of professionals. However, do not fret; there is some good news.

In early 2021, Amanda told me during one of our discussions that she had made the (wonderful, I might add) decision to share her strategies and resources for supporting struggling children in the shape of this book. I for one am delighted and relieved that we now have access to Amanda's resources, for guiding not just our children and pupils but also ourselves through these extraordinary times. Children, as far back as time began, have always faced trauma and adverse childhood experiences (ACEs). However, the extra layer of complexity brought about by the pandemic has thrown an additional, bulky and far from comfortable 'spanner in the works'. That just might be the understatement of the century.

Joking apart, anyone whose life and/or work involves looking after and raising children will have their own narrative of how the pandemic has changed or impacted on the behaviour of themselves and the children they know. Teachers and parents who have children's wellbeing at the centre of everything they do will surely be asking themselves, '*What can we do now to support children who are suffering due to loss and/or change?*'

Over the past 18 months, education authorities and local councils have responded in various ways to supporting children's wellbeing: some have issued wellbeing resources for families, schools and youngsters; others have offered guidelines to schools. Dr Pooky Knightsmith pushed for the Department of Education to fund Mental Health Leads in schools. All these are good starting points, but my questions remain:

- How do we help struggling children on a moment-by-moment, hour-by-hour, day-by-day basis to move forward?
- Do we have a plan?
- How do I help a child who I know is struggling now?

The answers are here, in comprehensive detail, in this resource. Educators and parents/carers can access practical, effective and tried-and-tested activities here, along with the author's own original materials, to start making a positive difference to their own and their children's/pupils' lives. The resources are refreshing, stimulating and pragmatic, and what is more, Amanda provides clear and easy-to-follow instructions for creating a positive environment for optimal results.

In this rich resource you will find that the author:

- Discusses what she has learnt from her work with children.
- Provides practical strategies and ideas to help children manage complex emotional situations.
- Presents easy-to-use lesson plans.
- Shares case studies.
- Gives theoretical background.

British researcher and Associate Professor of Psychobiology and Epidemiology, Dr Daisy Fancourt, of University College London (UCL), was recently able to prove that creativity has a profoundly positive effect on the brain and its ability to cope with trauma, depression, anxiety, emotional upheaval and stress. Her research focuses on the effects of social factors on health, including loneliness, social isolation, community assets, arts and cultural engagement and social prescribing. Perfectly in sync with these findings from UCL, Amanda has shared with us in this book, a range of powerful and effective creative activities that will help the grown up to support children through difficult times. A range of creative guided activities that the children will find fun and exciting awaits you in this book. These include designing a planet, making an alien puppet, building a space rocket and creating medals. The aim of this book is to empower adults – in turn to empower children. Amanda's mission is clear – and I can't think of a single educator who would disagree with it: to help children through the difficulties that loss and change present to us all; and, in turn, to become the heroes and heroines of their own stories. Children, who have already learnt the hard way that life is not always certain, can learn that loss and change *is* manageable with the right support and strategies. We can't go over loss and change; we can't go under it; 'Oh no, we've got to go through it', as Michael Rosen reminds us in *We're Going on a Bear Hunt* (1993). And it can be painful no doubt, but with care, the pain can be managed and eased.

Amanda also explores topics such as the notion of the physical and mental 'home' and what it means for us to be 'at home' with ourselves. She offers up ideas about how to tune in to our own internal radio and listen to ourselves, so that we can prepare ourselves for listening to our pupils and children. As educators it is vital that we don't ignore our own self-care and that we learn how to ready ourselves to help the adults of tomorrow to manage and monitor their own self-care too. Teachers are intelligent, articulate experts in people and their behaviours; and I truly believe that armed with these resources we will find ourselves with the capability to make a positive difference to the emotional wellbeing of pupils and children and prepare them for the lives that lie ahead of them. What I hope you take away from this book is the knowledge that we can make a positive difference for our pupils and children. What I know you will take away for sure is the inspiration to move forward, and the courage to take the 'right' next steps in your learning environment to avoid breakdowns and further trauma to the child and those around them.

Fiona Clark,
December 2021

Fiona Clark, also known as @spiralglass, has been a teacher for over two decades, and is the author of several books, including *A Practical Guide to Creative Writing in Schools: Seven Creative Writing Projects for Ages 8–14* (Routledge, 2021).

Preface

The COVID-19 pandemic has changed all of our lives, and amplified the challenges that we were facing before.

For children and young people who were already struggling with their mental health, because of traumatic experiences, social isolation, a loss of routine and a breakdown in formal and informal support, the pandemic has added another level of change.

When schools closed as part of necessary measures, children no longer had the sense of structure and stimulation that was provided by that environment. Their learning environment changed. They had less opportunity to be with their friends and get that social support that is essential for good mental health.

During lockdown, children faced numerous enforced changes and losses: home schooling, being isolated from teachers, no physical contact with their friends and grandparents, no playing outside their family homes, disrupted home routines as a result of parents working from home, cramped housing, strained family relationships, no transitions from one year group to the next. In vulnerable groups, these changes will have retraumatised children who were forced to live in domestic violent situations. Additionally, Covid produced 'death anxiety' and information overload. Children were likely to have experienced worry, anxiety and fear, and this can include the types of fears that are very similar to those experienced by adults, such as a fear of dying, a fear of their relatives dying or a fear of what it means to receive medical treatment.

Findings from Young Minds Covid-19 Autumn 2020 Survey Report

- 69% of respondents described their mental health as poor now that they are back at school; this has risen from 58% who described their mental health as poor before returning to school.
- 40% of respondents said that there was no school counsellor available to support students in their school.

- Only 27% had had a one-to-one conversation with a teacher or another member of staff in which they were asked about their wellbeing, by the time they completed the survey.
- Almost a quarter of respondents (23%) said that there was less mental health support in their school than before the pandemic, while only 9% agreed that there was more mental health support.

Learning to live with the impact of Covid-19 and all its variants has been described as the 'new normal'. Before we can accept this, we need to process the experiences, good and bad, that we have endured so that we can understand what our learning has been; what resources we have drawn on, who has helped us cope and what we are taking into this 'new normal' life.

While for many children school is their lifeline, a safe space, the reality during Covid is that teachers have been faced with a dual challenge: academic catch up from lockdown, and supporting children's mental health in light of their lockdown experience.

According to a new report by Barnardo's, New Term, New Challenges, New Opportunities, almost 90% of teachers agree the Covid-19 pandemic could have an impact on pupil's mental health.

The Institute of Public Policy Research study says fewer than half of state schools in England offer counselling for pupils on site in the wake of the coronavirus lockdown.

The risk, therefore, is that unless children are given the necessary mental health support, they will not reach their full potential. Barnardo's report on pandemic impact shows that schools cannot take on this challenge alone.

In view of the challenge teachers face, they need a practical toolkit which can be used inside and outside the classroom to help children tell their lockdown stories. This Toolkit can also be used by school mental health leads.

Aim of this book

The aim of this book is to give schools a therapeutic Toolkit based on the hero's journey, to use in the classroom to enable children to see themselves as the hero of their own story, and life, to reinstate a sense of optimism and self-empowerment in the face of the pandemic challenge and regain some control over their mental health and wellbeing. It builds on the concepts introduced in *Helping Children Cope with Loss and Change: A Guide for Professionals and Parents* (Seyderhelm, 2020).

A few years ago I read Maureen Murdock's book, *The Heroine's Journey* (1990). I was curious about the difference between this and the hero's journey, as set out by Joseph Campbell (2008). Both are about embarking on a quest, an adventure to find something that solves a problem. What I noticed about the heroes was that their journey appeared to be mostly an external one – finding an elixir, for example. For heroines, it was about reconnecting with the spiritually alive feminine Self, one who is actively engaged in the world, and who embraces the masculine principle as a mirror of herself.

To this we must now add another layer of examination.

> 'It would be wonderful for it to feel realistic for a woman to go on a hero's journey', says popular illustrator Alice Meichi Li. 'Alice in Wonderland and Dorothy in Oz as heroes only return to the status quo. When they win, they get to go home. Great you're home! Nothing's changed. It's not really a huge deal, you know?'
>
> (https://goodmenproject.com/featured-content/heros-journey-vs-heroines-journey-rewriting-privilege/)

Except it is a big deal. Returning home, or finding home, I believe is the purpose of the quest. To be able to locate ourselves fully, and to feel at home within ourselves, our skin, our family, community is the deal.

Homecoming is the central theme of this book, as in coming home to one's Self, which is the true purpose of taking the hero's journey. This might be after a period of upheaval, loss or change. We have certainly seen all of this during the pandemic, which started in 2019 and still continues. Home has been both a safe and unsafe place to be, depending on your circumstances. We were all told to 'stay at home' during 2020, and so the question has arisen: Who am I being at home, and how do I ground myself at home when all may be falling apart around me: domestic violence, abuse, economic poverty, mental health crises? And when the world outside is a threatening place, what happens to me when my home isn't safe? How do I then start to feel at home?

This moment in time has certainly made us rethink this question. And, it has made us think about our needs and how they are met, what's important, and what's irrelevant, what can we do without. What we can't do without is a place to call home within ourselves. A place where we can find comfort, joy, release from some of the external pressures. The traditional hero fights his demons and lives on. But in this story that we are living through, the journey destination is ourselves. We are fighting to learn how to be strong and resilient whatever the circumstances. When we narrow our focus like this it makes it easier somehow to find that soft place to fall.

The Toolkit contains a therapeutic story template for use in class groups as well as with individual children. This will enable teachers to incorporate the subject into Personal, Social, Health and Economic (PHSE) and Wellbeing lessons.

The Toolkit provides teachers with guidance around six therapeutic skill sets: trust, acceptance, witnessing, containing, active listening and becoming non-directive, all of which will help teachers contain children in the class and reduce the number of specialist referrals to mental health services that are already overwhelmed and unable to accept referrals.

Each chapter opens by asking a question, and the creative arts exercise is the tool you can use with the children to explore their answers.

Always remember that in all these exercises you are only attempting to facilitate bringing the children home to themselves, to that safe place within themselves that they can rely on, and trust. Call it an inner voice. Intuition. It is their own personal inner guidance that we want to encourage and support.

Nothing will change for children unless the environment around them also changes, and adapts to them, offers them hope and a glimpse that they are understood, not just taught, but understood. For this to happen schools need to embed a child-centred framework within their structure and system. They could start by learning how to help children tell their own stories, in a child's natural language of play.

Amanda Seyderhelm,
December 2021

References

Barnardo's (2020). 'New term. New challenges. New opportunities: Putting children's mental health at the heart of education'. August. Barnardo's Northern Ireland. Available at: https://www.barnardos.org.uk/sites/default/files/uploads/BarnardosNI-ChildrensMentalHealthAtTheHeartOfEducation.pdf[SC1] Challenges, New Opportunities.

Campbell, J. (2008). *The Hero with a Thousand Faces.* Novato, CA: New World Library.

Murdock. M. (1990).*The Heroine's Journey. Woman's Quest for Wholeness.* Boston: Shambhala Publications Inc.

Seyderhelm, A. (2020). *Helping Children Cope with Loss and Change: A Guide for Professionals and Parents.* Oxford: Routledge.

Young Minds (2020). 'Coronavirus: Impact on young people with mental health needs. Survey 3: Autumn 2020 – Return to school'. Young Minds. Available at: https://www.youngminds.org.uk/media/0h1pizqs/youngminds-coronavirus-report-autumn-2020.pdf.

Acknowledgements

My thanks and deepest gratitude go to:

- The families and schools who took part in my research which formed the basis of the case studies. All names have been changed to maintain confidentiality.
- Dennis McCarthy, Kate McKairt, Mooli Lahad and Lynne Souter-Anderson for your inspiring work in the creative therapeutic arts which continues to expand our conversation around the child being seen and heard in their own voice.
- Fiona Clark for not only writing the Foreword, but for also being a companion voice in this work.
- Clare Ashworth, my publisher at Routledge for being a strong and encouraging support throughout this book's evolution.
- My father, as always, for showing me that home, and being at home to myself, is the real gig.

Introduction

The hero

In my work with schools and families, the biggest challenge we face is a recognition that children don't talk directly about their feelings through language. They need to do this through their natural language of play.

The process of engaging the children through play needs to be facilitated by an adult, a play therapist, a parent, a pastoral lead or a mental health lead, who has been trained to use therapeutic play techniques. These include the use of therapeutic storytelling based on the hero's journey. However, it's not just about learning to engage with the child through the reading of the story, but also involves the quality of their listening and reflection. By actively listening and reflecting the adult learns where the child is struggling and what they need help with and can then make suggestions about how to support them.

Since I wrote my book *Helping Children Cope with Loss and Change* using therapeutic storytelling in 2020, children have endured enforced changes through the pandemic lockdowns. This has created an unprecedented amount of hardship, loss and grief for children and families, which has also amplified pre-existing inequalities in terms of poverty, social justice and racism. The lockdowns have been particularly challenging for children with special educational needs (SEN) and disabilities. In addition, according to Dr Nicole LePera (2021), while the ACEs (adverse childhood experiences) framework is useful, it doesn't tell us the full story of trauma. It fails to acknowledge the range of emotional and spiritual trauma, which are an outgrowth of consistently denying or repressing the needs of the authentic Self that so many of us have experienced: overt racism, discrimination and abuse, bigotry and bias that exist in the infrastructure of society. We live in a world that can be unsupportive and outright threatening – in the education system, prison system, health care system and most workplaces – we are existing in a near constant state of trauma.

This has implications in families where if parent figures have not healed or even recognised their unresolved traumas (something I write about in my first book, *Helping Children Cope with Loss and Change*), they cannot consciously navigate their own path in life, let alone act as trustworthy guides for someone else. According to Lindsay Gibson, a psychotherapist and the author of *Adult Children of Emotionally Immature Parents: How to Heal from Distant, Rejecting or*

DOI: 10.4324/9781003182009-1

Self-Involved Parents (2015), this lack of emotional connection in childhood leaves a 'gaping hole where true security might have been. The loneliness of feeling unseen by others is as fundamental a pain as physical injury.' This emotional loneliness continues into adulthood when we repeat these patterns of emotional avoidance, shut down and shaming.

Not recognising the upheaval children have been through during the pandemic, trying to urge, cajole and force them to 'catch up' academically before even attempting to understand what they might have lost or missed out on and the impact all of that has had on their emotional development is another trauma to add to this list.

Children need space and time, together with age-appropriate therapeutic tools, to help them make sense of, and express, their feelings about all of these unprecedented changes and traumas.

They need all of this to take place within a child-centred framework that allows them to direct their own discoveries with the support of a therapeutically trained adult.

This process is critical for healthy development and wellbeing, but without the right support it won't happen … This meaning-making process helps children to deal with their feelings, and alleviates suffering and long-term anxiety and depression.

Have you noticed how a child reacts if you ask them directly, 'How do you feel about Granny dying?' Most likely they will look away from you, change the subject or just shrug and say, 'Don't know'. These are typical reactions from children whose cognitive capacity has not yet developed to the stage where they can understand and verbally articulate their feelings, like adults.

The risk, therefore, is that children will feel isolated and misunderstood if no-one is speaking in their language. Problems they are struggling with will be suppressed and could end up leading to anxiety and depression. Children's natural language is play, and they are more likely to express their feelings indirectly through play and creativity.

Therapeutic storytelling is one such approach, which I introduced in *Helping Children Cope with Loss and Change*, and which I have developed further in this therapeutic Toolkit for schools. This approach uses metaphor to help bring about healing change in traumatic circumstances such as loss and bereavement. Therapeutic stories create sufficient coherence to facilitate talk about felt confusion or misunderstanding (Gersie, 1992).

The process is powerful in its simplicity. When a child identifies with the story character (for example, an animal losing its mother), and goes on the journey with the character, the child is able to process their traumatic emotions and feelings through the story character.

As a result of this, disturbed thoughts and feelings can be clarified with greater ease, and troubling memories are often worked through in a non-confrontational way for the child. This narrative cover gives children the chance to have their say about their loss without the challenge of committing themselves to an opinion.

The narrative structure of therapeutic stories closely follows the hero's journey, where the main character faces a challenge that he must learn how to overcome. Obstacles will appear along the way, and it's this central challenge which the child can relate to.

The story character learns life lessons and, importantly, how to draw on his own inner resources and those of the helpers who appear on his journey path. The story ends with the character winning his battle, and thus being transformed by the experience.

Rather than having a child read therapeutic stories alone, ideally, therapeutic stories should be read to a child, so that an adult can answer any questions. It's important to recognise that, if handled sensitively, a child's questions can lead to them opening up about their circumstances, but this must not be pushed.

Continuing with the animal example, I have heard children express sadness about an animal's loss, which is their indirect way of expressing their own sadness. They feel safe doing this, which means that the grieving process can begin on their terms.

What is therapeutic storytelling?

Stories use metaphor and imagery, a child's natural language for feeling (Sunderland, 2003, p. 2), to change the way we see our lives, and the world. Therapeutic stories connect us to ourselves, and each other, and help us find meaning, hope, resolution for life's problems.

Cantor (2007, p. 23) defines therapeutic storytelling as 'the process of constructing, co-constructing or otherwise utilising a narrative or anecdote with a client in the interest of achieving a therapeutic goal'.

A well-chosen therapeutic story can become a vital part of a child's healthy, emotional digestive system (Sunderland, 2003, p. xi) by getting to the heart of the matter, and giving children a 'safe distance' through metaphor to deal with their feelings. Readers or listeners project their own motives and emotions onto the characters featured in the story, be they human, animal, tree or a supernatural (imaginary) being. Catharsis and insight will complete the therapeutic impact of the story. The consequence of this healing process is diminished anxiety and increased self-esteem (Ayalon in Gersie, 1992, p. 17).

There are several therapeutic story frameworks used in play therapy, the most common of which is the hero's journey. The hero's journey was identified by the American scholar Joseph Campbell. This is a pattern of narrative that appears in drama, storytelling, myth, religious ritual and psychological development. It describes the typical adventure of the archetype known as The Hero, the person who goes out and achieves great deeds on behalf of the group, tribe or civilisation.

All frameworks have a beginning, middle and end which enables a child to learn and reflect upon their choices and intentions, practise and work out their own understanding and resolution. During their sessions, the child may return to the same story several times until they have played out their internal struggles and reached a resolution that makes sense to them. Through listening, and sometimes dramatising the story, the child goes on an emotional journey which results in a positive effect on their psychological and physical health (Greenberg and Stone, 1992 in Gersie, 1992, p.14). This encounter enables them to face down their fears, slay their demons within the safety of the story's metaphor and emerge victorious with new insights about inner resources. The play therapist listens and reflects back the child's experience, thereby strengthening the child's resolve. The teacher can learn to listen, reflect back and contain the child in the same way, by learning the therapeutic skills outlined in each chapter.

It's not possible for all children to have access to either play therapy or a school counsellor to engage in this creative therapeutic work. While for many children, school is their lifeline, a safe space, the reality is that teachers are faced with a dual challenge: academic catch up from lockdown, and supporting children's mental health in light of their lockdown experience. The risk, therefore, is that unless children are given the necessary mental health support, they will not reach their full potential.

Principles underpinning a child-centred approach

Underpinning the scaffolding of the therapeutic relationship are Axline's eight principles. While Axline's principles relate primarily to the therapeutic relationship, they also hold true for adults using a child-centred approach and building trust and rapport. The principles provide adult caregivers with the emotional scaffolding to hold on to, and return to, during this work. If they get lost or become unsure, these principles will guide them wisely.

Virginia Axline was a twentieth-century psychologist who pioneered the use of play therapy, which remains a popular method for treating children.

In 1964, Axline published a revolutionary and inspiring true story called *DIBS in Search of Self*. The book chronicled her therapeutic relationship with a 5-year-old boy who appeared withdrawn and uncommunicative. Though his parents suspected autism or severe mental retardation to be the cause of his behavior, Dibs emerged to find himself through play therapy over the course of several months. When he developed the necessary skills to show his true self to the world, Axline realised that he was a genius with an IQ of 168.

Axline worked extensively to develop her non-directive approach to play therapy, in which she identified eight distinct, core principles (Axline, A. 1969):

1. *Establishing rapport*: The therapist must develop a warm, friendly relationship with the child, in which good rapport is established as soon as possible.
2. *Accepting the child completely*: The therapist must accept the child exactly as they are.
3. *Establishing a feeling of permissiveness*: The therapist must establish a feeling of permissiveness in the relationship so that the child feels completely free to express their feelings.
4. *Recognition and reflection of feelings*: The therapist is alert to recognise the feelings the child is expressing and reflects back those feelings in such a manner that the child gains insight into their behaviour.
5. *Maintaining respect for the child*: The therapist maintains a deep respect for the child's ability to solve their own problems if given the opportunity. The responsibility to make choices and to institute change is the child's.
6. *The child leads the way*: The therapist does not attempt to direct the child's actions or conversation in any manner. The child leads the way. The therapist follows.

7. *Therapy cannot be hurried*: The therapist does not attempt to hurry the therapy along. It is a gradual process and is recognised as such by the therapist.
8. *The value of limitations*: The therapist establishes only those limitations that are necessary to anchor therapy to the world of reality and to make the child aware of their responsibility in the relationship.

Aim of this book

The aim of this book is to give schools a therapeutic storytelling toolkit to use in the classroom to enable children to tell their lockdown stories, and regain some control over their mental health and wellbeing. It builds on the concepts introduced in *Helping Children Cope with Loss and Change: A Guide for Professionals and Parents*.

The 'Toolkit' follows the hero's journey template for use in class groups as well as with individual children. This will enable teachers to incorporate the subject into PHSE and wellbeing lessons.

The Toolkit provides teachers with guidance around six therapeutic skill sets: trust, acceptance, witnessing, containing, active listening and becoming non-directive, all of which will help teachers contain children in the class and reduce the number of specialist referrals to mental health services, which are already overwhelmed and unable to accept referrals.

References

Axline, V. (1964). *DIBS In Search of Self*. Middlesex: Penguin Books.

Axline, V. (1969). *Play Therapy*. New York: Ballantine Books.

Gersie, A. (1992). *Storymaking in Bereavement: Dragons Fight in the Meadow*. London: Jessica Kingsley Publishers.

Gibson, L.C. (2015). *Adult Children of Emotionally Immature Parents: How to Heal from Distant, Rejecting, or Self-involved Parents*. Oakland, CA: New Harbinger Publications.

LePera, N. (2021). *How to Do the Work, Recognise Your Patterns, Heal from the Past and Create Your Self*. London: Orion Spring.

The Toolkit

Introduction

To prepare for working with a child, there are three areas to focus on:

- Centring your mind, body and spirit.
- Your relationship with the child.
- The physical environment where the storytelling takes place.

Centring your mind, body and spirit

Just as you would prepare your body to run a marathon, so it's important to prepare yourself and the children for a hero's journey. To get yourself in the best shape, there are three elements I like to focus on:

- Attuning to your stress signals.
- Becoming safely embodied.
- Containment.

Attuning to your stress signals

For both self-care purposes and session preparation, I recommend completing an exercise I call 'The drawing check-in' which will help you to become attuned to your stress signals. This will help you to develop a good sense of how your body communicates to you when it is overwhelmed.

Before I begin any session I do three things: I remind myself how the previous session ended, reflect on session notes and ask (invoke) what I need as preparation for the next session. This helps me to prepare and link into the next session by remembering the themes and tone of the child's story. I find it helpful to have prepared a structure for holding the child which creates a space for vulnerability. An invocation – ritual at the start of each session provides such a structure. I use the drawing check-in to ground us in the present. This helps the child leave behind what

DOI: 10.4324/9781003182009-2

has been affecting them before they entered the session. It creates an atmosphere of safety and helps me to attune to the child which, in turn, allows them to open their emotional tap.

The drawing check-in

One of the most useful tools that I use during training professionals is called the drawing check-in. Teachers, social workers and therapists have learned to incorporate this tool into their professional practice because it is a way for them to reflect on their feelings. The exercise also helps them to reduce stress and anxiety because creating the drawing connects them to the right-hand side of their brain, where their emotions and feelings are. The drawing itself functions as a container – you literally draw out your feelings onto the page and voilà, you will immediately feel lighter, ready to start your day.

When you practise the drawing check-in every day, you will start to create a dialogue with yourself that gives you feedback about your mind (racing thoughts), body (sweating, breathing difficulties) and feelings (sadness and fear).

Remember, we can't think our way out of anxiety with the same mindset that put us there. We shift our mindset by connecting with the story part (the right-hand side) of our brain, and let the drawings tell us how to reset our calm and make the connection.

When you are practising the drawing check-in for self-care and invocation purposes, follow the instructions below.

FOR SELF-CARE

This exercise is best done in the morning, before going to school, which will help you start the day feeling connected to yourself.

All you need to do this exercise is a small Tupperware box filled with coloured crayons and some white A4 paper. I like to include different textures of crayons so that if I feel like scrawling or making heavy marks on the page, I select the oil pastels which work better than a light pencil.

Set aside 30 minutes to complete this exercise. With practice you will be able to do it in 15 minutes. It is a great way to start the day. Sit somewhere quiet where you will not be disturbed. Turn your phone off. Ask yourself: How am I feeling right now? Select your crayons and draw a picture which represents your feeling. Try not to critique yourself, you aren't creating perfection, just a picture of how you feel. Remember, whatever you produce is OK, it's a reflection of how you feel. When you've finished drawing your picture, take a few moments to look at and reflect on it, and write one word on the drawing which describes your feeling. You are literally meeting yourself on the page, so whatever shows up, just acknowledge it. You will be amazed how powerful this exercise is over time. You can keep the drawings if you want to but it's fine if you want to immediately dispose of them.

To reflect on your image, use these three prompts, and write in your journal.
Your daily prompts:

1. IMAGE

    What does this image tell me about myself and my situation today?

2. MY THREE WORDS

    What do my words mean to me? Can I see a connection between them and my image?

3. CHECK-IN

    What are the actions I need to take based on these words?

STORYTELLING PREPARATION

When you practise the drawing check-in as preparation for a heroic storytelling session with a child, you give the child the opportunity to pause and settle, gather themselves in preparation for the story session. You will also glean valuable insight into their state of mind and feelings. This will be easier, less confrontational than asking them directly how they are feeling.

There are four steps involved in the storytelling:

1. Invite the child to choose three coloured crayons from the box.
2. Read the story – 'Hemi and the Whale' – to them.
3. Ask the child to draw an image after hearing the story.
4. Ask the child to write one word on the image.

Hemi and the Whale

Once there was a small boy called Hemi who lived near the sea. Every morning he woke up early and went down to the seashore to explore and look at the sea. Every day there was something different to look at, it was always changing and he loved it.

One morning, there was something very different on the beach … very different and very large. It made Hemi's heart flip over. It was a whale! There it was, lying on the sand so still.

Hemi ran over to look at the whale thinking it was dead but he saw the blowhole open and close and realised the whale was still breathing. So, he ran back up to the house to call his grandmother: 'Granny, Granny, get water quick. There's a whale on the beach!' He ran and got buckets and started filling them with water but they were very heavy and it took all his strength not to spill the water on the way.

Meanwhile his grandmother, looking out the window, saw what was happening and called his grandfather. His grandfather called the neighbour and the neighbour called another neighbour and that neighbor called another and ….

Suddenly there was a whole group of people running up and down the beach carrying buckets of water trying to keep the whale wet until the incoming tide could float it back out to sea again. Someone brought bed sheets to cover the whale and help keep its skin moist.

Finally the tide came in and began to wash up against the mighty animal. Hemi was right by its head when the whale opened one unblinking, liquid, black eye. 'Hold on, whale', said Hemi. 'You will be home soon.'

Then everyone worked together to support the whale. Some pulled on the sheets to steer the beast, and others pushed from behind, struggling in the foamy water and the wet sand.

Finally, they felt the life come back into the whale. Its body shuddered, and it took one massive breath through its blowhole, and then blew out again. It nosed down into the sea, and slipped off the sheets and helping hands, and a big cheer went up as it flicked its tail and began to swim back out to sea.

Hemi stayed on the seashore long after everyone else had gone, watching the waves and scanning the horizon for his whale. Finally his grandmother came down and put her arm around him. She said, 'I am really proud of you, Hemi.' Then they slowly walked back to the house together.

(Story sourced through Zakheni Arts Therapy
Foundation, South Africa,
https://www.facebook.com/zakhenitransformativearts)

Becoming safely embodied

Learning how to become safely embodied and stop yourself becoming emotionally numb by being able to be fully present in the moment will help you to cope more ethically and empathically when you are with a child who is unpacking traumatic experiences in their heroic story.

Mindfulness is an accepted practice for calming and regulating a frazzled, anxious, racing mind. Ruby Wax's book, *A Mindfulness Guide for Survival* (2021) is a useful workbook which explains the five pillars of mindfulness: insight, stress reduction, emotional awareness, presence and kindness or compassion. As she explains, thoughts don't stop. What can change with the practice of mindfulness is our relationship to them.

Dr Tina Rae has an exercise called 'Mindful breathing-blowing bubbles' in her book, *A Toolbox of Wellbeing*, which is an activity you can use yourself as well as with anxious children.

Mindful breathing-blowing bubbles
The Bubble Blowing Technique is one of the best mindful breathing techniques for young children. Give each child a small container of bubbles so they can practise blowing bubbles with a wand. They will learn quickly that if they blow too hard or too fast, the bubble will burst before it has time to take shape. By blowing slowly and with purpose, they can blow a perfect bubble.

I teach a simple technique to be fully present which I have found useful in my clinical practice, and I call this 'The ONE click method'.

This was originally taught to me by my meditation teacher, Lee Everett, many years ago, and it is the quickest way of being present to oneself and others. Over the years it has enabled me to bring my busy mind back to my present situation. What can happen in stressful situations is the mind goes into 'fight or flight' mode which means that we lose our connection to our rational thinking as our body adrenalin rises to an unhealthy level and we can overreact to a situation. This overreaction is something that we would not usually do, but at the time of reaction we can't see this, all we can feel is fear, so we 'take off' and can sound unreasonable and not ourselves. You will recognise this moment before 'take off' because your body might feel hot or flushed. What we want is to be able to stop ourselves from reaching this 'take off' point, and we can do that by using the ONE click method.

The ONE click method

If you know that you are going to be entering a potentially difficult situation that might make your blood pressure rise (!), I want you to 'take 5 minutes' before entering that situation and use the ONE click method.

Find a quiet spot to take your 5 minutes. Loos are everywhere and I usually find this is the quietest place where I can be alone with my thoughts. No-one will argue with you saying you need to use the loo! Go into the cubicle and close the door. Sit down on the closed loo seat. You will find that the doors of the loo function to shut out all the noise that might be trying to overwhelm your brain. Close your eyes and take a few moments to slow your breathing down. Breathe in through your nose and out through your mouth five times. You should start to feel calmer just from doing this. Open your eyes. Think about leaving the loo and entering the meeting calmly, and at this point raise your pen writing hand until it's at eye level and CLICK your fingers once, firmly. You should be able to hear the click clearly. In that CLICK feel yourself being fully present in your body. Stand up and stretch your arms up. Feel the tension leaving your body and being replaced with strength and energy. You are ready to leave the loo and enter your situation feeling calm and present.

Repeat this exercise as often as you like. You will eventually reach the stage where you don't have to use the loo to use the ONE click method because you will be able to simply visualise yourself doing this which will instantly bring you back into your body and present situation.

Containment

Teachers are containing children, stories and themselves all day, five days a week, which can be exhausting. Sometimes if we don't contain ourselves enough we can get a sense of losing ourselves, which just means we may start to feel disconnected from ourselves. This is when situations can feel distorted. We might misconstrue or misunderstand something a child or parent says to us, we might overreact, start taking things personally, etc. I have found that one way to help reconnect you to your true self and find a comfortable sense of containment again is through painting and creating a series of what I call 'Quest paintings'. Again, this is an exercise I use in all my training courses and in my own self-care practice and which can be completed in an hour. Once you are familiar with the set up and process of this exercise you can shorten it according to the time you have available. I recommend doing the long version once a month for a few months before trying the shortened version. To do the shortened version you will need to have the resources for this exercise ready to use. I keep the resources in a small plastic box and find a fold-out gardening table which extends and is the best surface to use. I keep this folded up when not in use, and it takes two minutes to unfold and extend ready to use. I wipe it clean afterwards and it doesn't matter if paint gets splattered on it.

The image I use for this exercise is a labyrinth or maze. The labyrinth is a symbol of the Quest in its many forms. The Quest is for what has been lost, one's own soul or essential Self. There is only one path which leads eventually to numerous experiences where one is forced to make constant choices. This endless confrontation with new experiences and choices constitutes the labyrinth within which we must search for meaning and direction and ultimately find the Path of Liberation which leads out of the labyrinthian life (Eversole, 2012; Seyderhelm, 2020).

The original inspiration for this painting practice came from Suzette Clough's Visual Medicine technique she calls 'no brush painting'.

What you are going to do

Paint 20 small paintings over a 30-minute period.

What you will need:

- 1 pack of Indian Khadi paper available at: www.khadi.com.
- 1 plastic container to use as a water bucket to wet your paper.
- Jam jars, each one filled with the primary colour paints mixed to a thickish pouring consistency.
- A single A3 plastic sheet.
- A table mat to use as a paint mixing board.

In this picture you can see the individual 'stations' set up with Khadi paper, water buckets and jam jars filled with different colour paints. Some of the Quest paintings are visible on the large plastic sheet set up for the group. These paintings were created in the course of an afternoon and provided rich insights for all participants into their individual processes. After completing the exercise we sat in a circle and reflected on the feelings that arose from the exercise; some participants wrote words on the back of their paintings to 'claim' them, others sat quietly, reflecting privately on what had arisen.

It's helpful at the end of the reflective stage to identify the relevance of the message and how it relates to your current (or past) situation. If there is something you are struggling with, a relationship or a situation at work or at home, this exercise will provide you with insights into what you need to see or learn from it.

Taking it a step further, you can select one or several paintings, paste them inside your journal and write in your journal about them. Over time, this helps you to stay engaged with your inner guidance of intuition and sensitivity.

I understand if you feel this may not be for you if you have never enjoyed painting. All I would say is that I have seen many, many practitioners and participants of this exercise approach it with hesitation and end up with incredulous joy – they can't quite believe how powerful and revealing it is, in a helpful way, so I encourage you to give it a try.

NO BRUSH PAINTING METHOD

Place the plastic sheet on the floor or table. Set your table mat on the floor or table, in front of you. Fill your water bucket with water. Place your Khadi papers (you should have 20 small pieces about A5 size) in the water. Shake and then uncap your jars of

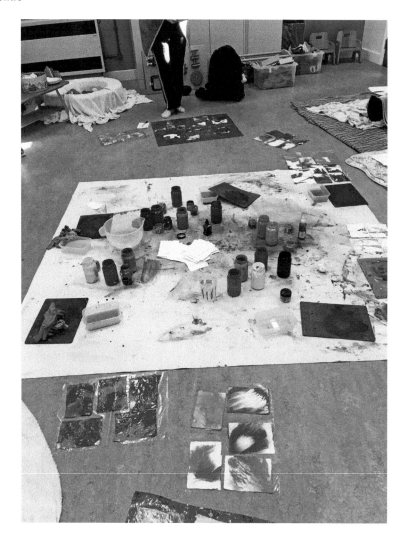

Figure I.1 Group training to support self-containment and reflective practice in the Family Support Team at Leicester City Council, showing the Quest painting set-up.

paint. Select three colours and pour a large blob of paint onto the table mat. Select a piece of wet paper and touch the edges of the paint with this. With your free hand pick up the table mat so that the paint moves onto the paper and just play with the movement of the paint. When you have enough paint on the paper, put the table mat down and spend time moving the paper around, watching the wet paint drizzle and dribble around the paper. Notice the shapes and feelings that are aroused in you while you are doing this. When you are happy with the painting, set it down on the plastic sheet in front of you. Repeat this exercise until you have completed all 20 paintings.

I like to play music while completing this exercise as this can change your mental state so that you are more receptive to the colours and textures, feeling the paint on your hands, noticing how getting messy makes you feel! Some people love this and others don't. Just notice how you feel.

Take 15 minutes to write in your journal what the experience felt like.
Things to pay attention to: patterns and themes which recur in the 20 paintings. Some people notice that once they have sat looking at the paintings and reflecting on their meaning, suddenly an idea of what they are about will come to them. This is important information to pay attention to because it is coming from your higher self, what is sometimes called your spiritual Self. This can give real significance to the whole Quest, and you may find that the meaning of the paintings stays with you for several days. I have had pupils feel quite transformed by doing this exercise. Old, stubborn patterns of thinking and behaviour can shift quickly while doing this exercise, so don't be surprised if you find yourself suddenly making connections. This is what we want! Write it all down in your journal.

Your relationship with the child

After parents and caregivers, a teacher is usually the most significant other adult in a young child's life, with the power to influence and engage that child, to help them grow and develop, build courage and resilience. All of this is done as well as engaging within the context of the educational task (Salmon, 1995).

Developmental psychology shows us that the child's self-image is internalised from significant others. The teacher's ability to listen actively, respond empathically, provide consistency and establish clear boundaries can all help the child feel secure within this relationship. You help the child develop a more positive Self by showing that both their anxieties and their story have been, as Winnicott (1960, p. 240) puts it, 'held in mind'. This holding in mind needs to be made explicit to the pupil and it is the practical ways of doing this that underpin my therapeutic storytelling approach. For example, by using active listening skills the teacher can show the children they are aware of the children's personal anxieties. Reflective comments made verbally or in writing on the children's work are used to show them that the feelings expressed in their story have been thought about. With the security the children receive from knowing the teacher has them in mind, they become less preoccupied with their anxieties and are able to focus on the educational task (Waters, 2004).

The six skills you will need to *decode* a child's hero's journey

These skills are trust, acceptance, witnessing, containing, active listening and becoming non-directive. The skills are covered at the end of each chapter.

The physical environment where the storytelling takes place

Given that the story will be unfolding over a period of weeks, sometimes months, it's important that you have in place your scenery which will scaffold the storytelling.

Imagine you are working in a theatre company. The play unfolds on stage in the context of scenery, which provides a backdrop as well as the foundation for the storytelling. It holds the story. In some cases, the scenery wraps its arms around the stage, enfolding you but, as an audience, you get to see into the storytelling, to bear witness, there is space for the projection of voices and the audience's response. It's this type of atmosphere and structure you are going to create for your heroic story-telling. Unless you have the luxury of leaving this scenery in place permanently, you will need to be able to easily pack and unpack this scenery before each storytelling session. I recommend keeping this in a small, plastic box.

Over the years that my practice has evolved, I have worked to get my scenery to fit into this plastic box: crayons, paper and a story. I should say that it is the practice that has shaped the size of the box, and not the other way around. In other words I haven't compromised or scrimped on the scope or scale of the scenery. This is an important point. Don't let the size of your physical space limit or determine the shape of your scenery. That is putting the cart before the horse, so to speak. I have set up this scenery in large, physical training spaces as well as on Zoom. Think about what scenery you want and go from there. When your thinking is complete, then is the time to consider scaling it back so that it fits. But if you approach this exercise the other way around, you will short-circuit your creative energy, and you won't fully extend your vision. The children will feel that limitation. If all you have to work in is a cupboard, make sure that your thinking isn't as narrow as that space. A huge vision can be communicated in a tiny space. However, if you allow the size of the space to dictate your vision, you will end up cutting corners, and shoe-boxing your vision.

Don't do that.

Reference

Waters, T. (2004). *Therapeutic Storywriting: A Practical Guide to Developing Emotional Literacy in Primary Schools*. Abingdon: Routledge.

Chapter 1

The Call

Introduction

The hero (child) is faced with something that makes them begin their adventure. This might be a problem or a challenge they need to face and overcome. It might be finding themself in a new situation where they need to make emotional and physical adjustments to settle in. In general they must make a choice about whether to undertake the adventure. Sometimes school staff become aware that the child is facing 'the Call' only when the child goes into some kind of crisis. Behaviour changes and becomes more problematic. This is the child's cry for help. They are flagging up that they feel overwhelmed, and want help with processing their feelings. They want you to be a witness. Sometimes the Call is forced onto the child.

This case study looks at the Call in relation to adapting to home being without a parent, a mother, and the challenge of what it means to find 'home' in that context. To be at home in oneself, and not just in a physical sense of having a room of your own. To feel accepted unconditionally.

Home is both a physical place where children live, eat and sleep and a mental and emotional place they inhabit. When they feel secure and safe in their relationship with these spaces as well as their carers, these spaces cohabit in a way that enables the child to thrive.

We have seen during the 2020 pandemic how the concept of being at home has changed. For bereaved children, any changes which impact their feelings of security may also trigger their feelings of being abandoned. For these children, some of whom have also experienced high levels of early life disruption, we need to be particularly aware of any changes in their behaviour. Our response to any changes needs to be driven by a child-centred, age-appropriate intervention such as therapeutic play. In the following case study you will see how an understanding of what home meant took time to fully appreciate. I believe the intervention of play therapy shortened the time factor because the child felt heard and understood during this process.

DOI: 10.4324/9781003182009-3

For the child the Call was multidimensional: Who am I now without my Mother? Am I accepted as I am? Am I loved? These are questions the child is asking you indirectly. It's likely that the depth of their Call will be expressed through metaphor in younger children. When this happens, learn to decode that metaphor. The home may not appear literally as a house, it may look like a cave, a cupboard, a boat. There are many ways in which home can be expressed. Whatever the metaphor is, know that it holds the key to what's inside the child's inner world. It's full of meaning.

Is the Call about fitting in, being accepted or being loved? Remember that self-esteem and confidence improve when the child feels unconditionally accepted and understood. So your activities need to be based around this.

I have found that repetition is important when working with bereaved children. They need to repeat activities until they have 'got' it.

The place you want to reach in the Call stage is to have established trust. You want to ensure that the child knows you are a safe companion for their journey with you into their story. If they are going to open up to you, they need to feel safe, and this won't happen unless you have built trust between you. This is the most important tool in your toolkit. Making the time to create trust will save you time in the end. Without trust the child will resist the intervention, be unwilling to go deep, and keep you at arm's length. It will not succeed because they will withhold their story and you will not be able to build a connection with them. This is the equivalent of making sure you have all the equipment and resources for a journey you are about to undertake. If you set off half-rigged, you will most likely fall at the first hurdle. When you are helping a child tell their story, it is the trust between you that will enable the child to carry on, in spite of the hurdles. You are the bridge. The creative tools are helpful in terms of enabling the child to express their feelings, and cross the bridge, but it is the relationship between you and the child that will determine the quality of meaning making and shared understanding. Trust is important at each stage in the journey, and the ideal place we are aiming to reach is where the child feels safe enough within themselves, to feel at home and to trust themselves, to continue on their journey without you.

RS – where is *my* 'home'?

Case summary

This is a review of three drawings made by a 7-year-old girl called RS, referred to me following the death of her mother. I saw RS for 12 individual sessions of non-directed play therapy at Great Dalby Primary School, Leicestershire. These drawings (see Figures 1.1, 1.2 and 1.3) were made over the first eight sessions, two of which were house-tree-person (HTP) projected drawings, the third was a spontaneous client-generated drawing.

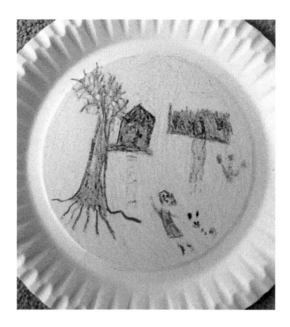

Figure 1.1 HTP drawing 1.

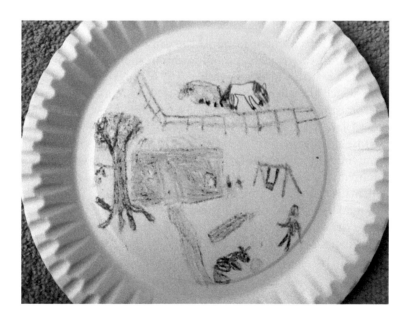

Figure 1.2 HTP drawing 2.

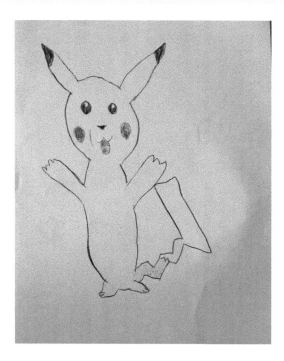

Figure 1.3 Spontaneous drawing 3.

My review takes into account not only the drawings as objects, but also as an embodiment of the transference and echo of the unconscious aspects of the therapeutic relationship (Schaverien, 1991, p. 65). The paper is a safe space onto which the client's projections are placed, and the symbols and images become the containers of emotions, which allows their feelings to be expressed (Allan, 1988, p. 22). These drawings were subjective creations, and therefore my evaluation of them will focus on the pictures' psychological content, and 'feeling' (Furth, 1988, p. 33). The drawings were made using coloured Crayola markers which gave the pictures a grainy, indistinct look, which overall made me feel uncertain, and shaky. The HTP drawings were made on white paper plates, symbolising the mandala and the spontaneous drawing was made on white A4 paper. My review refers to the work and principles of Gregg M. Furth (1988), John Buck (1948), and Joy Schaverien (1991).

The drawings

Created by John Buck in 1948, HTP is a projective drawing technique designed to give the therapist information about an individual's 'sensitivity, maturity, flexibility, efficiency, degree of personality integration, and interaction with the environment' (Furth, 1988, p. 24).

HTP drawing 1 (Figure 1.1)

Overwhelmed, grounded, shaky and lost are the feelings evoked by this HPT drawing. RS drew this picture during session 6, one year after her mother's death. RS was very close to her mother, and since her death had slept with several fictional soft toy creatures called Pokemon, particularly a character called Pikachu (drawn here as the small yellow character holding onto the girl's hand), which were gifts from her mother. Culturally, Pokemon has become a global game phenomenon amongst young children. Conversation about Pikachu dominated RS's sessions. I therefore felt it important to review this symbol, showing how RS transferred her feelings of loss about her mother onto the Pikachu object, and into the 'picture within the frame' (Schaverien, 1991, p. 65).

The Pokemon characters are trained to fight by humans, and can take on the traits and feelings of their trainers. Pikachu has suffered some betrayals or letdowns in his past which has led him to be closed-minded and unwelcoming of others. Until rapport and trust were established between us, RS was well defended and cautious. Over the course of the sessions, our relationship developed so she spoke to me through Pikachu and her drawings about her feelings.

Schaverien (1991, p. 63) says the art object, like the scapegoat, becomes embodied, empowered and is subsequently disposed of, and that this may result in a resolution of some inner conflict. By containing her story within the picture, RS was able to contain aspects of her grieving process and start the letting-go process of Pikachu, as the transference between us deepened, and she realised I was going to return to see her each week. I was constantly aware of the loss of my mother during these sessions, and this 'picture within the frame' of our therapeutic relationship held and protected RS and me from the potentially overwhelming nature of the unconscious content of the picture, and the transference (Schaverien, 1991, p. 66).

The house is a symbol of the core Self. There are two houses in this picture, a tree house attached to the tree and a separate house with a yellow roof, which might suggest the split and separation caused by the death of RS's mother. A roof is associated with memories. Yellow may suggest an emphasis on things of a spiritual or intuitive nature, something of great value, as well as being associated with a precarious life situation (Furth, 1988, p. 98). I am struck by the three yellow images: ladder, Pikachu and roof, which evoke feelings of hope and expectation, and I wonder if these might also reflect RS's feelings of warm memories of her mother.

The house with the brown interior shows no signs of life at all, and feels like it's a big mess. Furth (1988, p. 98) says brown can be associated with nourishment, in touch with nature and the terrestrial, as well as rot or decay, or a struggle to overcome destructive forces and return to a healthy state, and I wonder if the mess symbolises the messy family grief. There is a faint door outlined in black and a single black window, both of which look open because I can see the brown mess inside. In spite of the path leading to the front door, I feel blocked from entering, and unwelcome. This feeling is in contrast to the tree house ladder which has distinct steps to climb up into and down from the tree house. The tree house has a red door with a black door knob, and a small window with blue bars. These details, together with the close proximity of the tree house to the tree makes me feel lively, and curious about what's inside the tree house!

The tree symbolises a person's security, and here the roots look deeply grounded, but the way one root is extending towards the girl evokes feelings of loss for me, perhaps symbolising RS's loss of her mother. The tree has a strong trunk, with many branches and green leaves.

The person symbolises the ego. The person's body, which looks like a girl's body, appears to be leaning backwards as she points towards the ladder, as if she is going to climb up the yellow ladder into the tree house, taking those memories with her through her attachment to Pikachu. In the picture the girl is standing next to Pikachu. She appears to have two arms, two legs and feet, and is wearing red shoes. She looks as if she is standing on tiptoe, which reminds me of how RS is tiptoeing around her grieving father. Her hands are indistinct, and she appears to be pointing or waving with one arm, and holding onto Pikachu with the other. She is wearing a pink dress, with something pink in her hair, which reminds me of the pink butterfly RS wears in her hair which was a gift from her mother, and might suggest she has taken on her mother's role with her father. I feel alarmed looking at her, especially her black eyes and mouth. Black may indicate or symbolise the unknown, and feels here as if it's associated with the darkness and emptiness of the bereaved state. The Pikachu, itself a stuffed toy, is dead, and yet very much alive for RS in the way that he represents her mother, and embodies her transferred loss.

The green background and three pink flowers make me feel hopeful, and might suggest a healthy ego and body; growth or a newness of life, as in the healing process (Furth, 1988, p. 98).

Here, RS has chosen to draw within the mandala shape, and reflect her inner and outer worlds. The picture serves as the Other, the object through which RS's inner world can be seen.

HTP drawing 2 (Figure 1.3)

Happiness and peacefulness are the feelings evoked by this picture.

The tree house in HTP2 looks larger than it did in HTP1, and makes me wonder if the two houses in HTP1 have been combined to form a larger house. If so, this new formation could also represent some kind of internal integration for RS. This roof looks golden yellow, which to Furth (1988, p. 98) suggests an emphasis on things of a spiritual or intuitive nature, and something of great value. To me this roof feels like it's crowning the house, with a life-force energy. There are two windows with red curtains and some white space, and the door has some green markings.

However, I feel very sad looking at this house. The windows are lopsided, reminding me of a sad face, and the brown mess still covers the house. The appearance of animals and the black shape in the bottom of the picture (RS's guinea pig) make me feel less lonely, and the swing and slide suggest evidence of, and an opportunity for, playfulness. The fence around the animals makes me feel there is a barrier somewhere between the animals, the house and playfulness, yet the fence also provides a form of containment for the animals. This paradox makes me feel ambivalent, and I wonder what that ambivalence might be suggesting. The back-to-back positioning of the two fenced-in animals makes me feel some kind of opposing energetic force, which might relate to messiness and synthesis, and the white body of the black-haired animal makes me feel hopeful as this might be a sign of a new lightness coming into RS's life.

The tree has grown closer to the tree house and there is a narrow gap now between the two, with some pink blossoms, perhaps reflecting the blossoming taking place within RS and within our therapeutic relationship, and a narrow individuation process.

The person looks like a boy and appears to be sitting or partially lying on his side. He has arms and legs, but no feet or hands. His facial features are indistinct. He looks lost, and I feel lonely looking at him, separated from the animals by the fence. I feel anxious about him sitting alone.

The second HTP drawing makes me feel like RS's world has expanded a little.

Spontaneous drawing 3

I have placed this drawing within Allan's (1988, pp. 20–63) 'Initial' stage because it shows an image that reflects RS's internal world.

Startled, wary and alarmed are the feelings evoked by this drawing. This drawing was made on white A4 paper during session 8, after HTP1 and HTP2.

The Pikachu's red tongue is sticking out in a rude and aggressive gesture. Pikachu has been trained to fight, and in this drawing his tongue signals hostility towards me, the viewer. The colour red may signal an issue of vital, 'burning' significance, surging emotions or danger (Furth, 1988, p. 98). His two red cheeks suggest he is flushed with anger and heat. His outstretched arms make me feel ambivalent: I'm not sure whether this posture means he is welcoming me, or getting ready to fight and be defensive. Does he want a hug, or a battle ...? I'm not sure, but his pointed black ears signal alertness. His squiggly tail frightens me. Overall I feel threatened by this picture. At first glance he looks like a sweet character, but closer inspection makes me feel uncomfortable, especially his black, glassy eyes. The size of his ears is disproportionately large compared with his other facial features, and make me wonder if he is hyper-vigilant, always attuning himself to other people, something RS was doing with her Father for whom she felt responsible and concerned about because he was not coping well with his grief. RS assumed a care-taking role with him, and got up early in the morning before school to make her father a cup of tea and a biscuit, which she took to him on a tray. If her father was ill or had a headache, she became anxious, and talked about him during her sessions, perhaps fearful of the possibility that he might also die and leave her alone.

RS started inhabiting the Pokemon world more and more, with her friends, making up games during break play times, and out of school time taking him with her on a school trip. Here Pikachu looks static, frozen, lifeless, with a trapped-in-the-headlights look about him, which mirrored how I felt being with RS in the play room, trapped in that space with her grief and loss. The size and scale of this image reflect the importance of this character in RS's life.

Jung (Schaverien, 1991, p. 21) understood from his own experience, and from observing his patients create them, that making pictures was a useful method of getting in touch with the healing aspects of the unconscious. These three drawings show the progression RS made in her healing.

Theoretical background: understanding mark making in children's drawings

In pictures and drawings, we see, as Jung emphasised, the unification of the conscious and unconscious mind (Furth, 1988, p. 24). Every mark in a child's drawing (lines, colours, shapes, shading, emphasis and their relationship to one another) is significant. As play therapists, we can discover and illuminate meaning for ourselves by examining the picture's marks, symbols, energy and relationships, although Furth (1988, p. 16) cautions us to look at the drawing with no preconceived ideas and with an openness so we don't easily project our own psychology onto the drawing. Don't fall into this trap! I want to emphasise the importance of following his guidance when you are looking at children's drawings. Invite the children to tell you about their drawings and listen to what they tell you, and for references to their feelings. Be careful not to analyse their drawings and point out what you see until they claim it for themselves. If you do this, you may be short-circuiting the child sharing insightful information about their world view. It's possible that they see something entirely different from your adult eye. Their interpretation, if they give you one, is the one to reflect back to them. You aren't being an art critic here, you are an active witness to their unfolding story.

Research studies have shown that anxieties, conflicts and attitudes are often communicated in the drawings by unique signs and symbols, and vary according to client and timeframe. At best, there may be several characteristics that consistently indicate emotional problems. Therefore, meaningful diagnoses cannot and should not be made from a single sign; rather, the total drawing, as well as combinations of indicators, must always be included when analysing the drawing (Malchiodi, 2007, p. 24).

Different theories on colour interpretation do not always agree on specific meanings, but theorists agree that colours can symbolise certain feelings, moods, even the tone of a relationship. Furth (1988, p. 98) says colours don't tell the picture's story, they amplify what the objects and action within the picture have to say. In my review I refer to Furth's colour interpretations.

Lesson plan: draw a house-tree-person

The exercise I have chosen for this lesson expands on the concept of home and invites children to draw a picture of a house, a tree and a person. It is also known as the House-Tree-Person (HTP Projective Test, which is used to explore a person's cognitive, emotional and social functioning. The drawings are all made on a paper plate. In Oriental art and religion, the mandala is a symbol of the unified Self and the Universe (Furth, 1988, p. 82).

In play therapy, a child's drawings are seen not only as objects, but also as an embodiment of the transference and echo of the unconscious aspects of the therapeutic relationship (Schaverien, 1991, p. 65). The paper used for drawing is a safe space onto which the client's projections are placed, and the symbols and images become the containers of emotions, which allows the child's feelings to be expressed (Allan, 1988, p. 22). The drawings the children make will be their subjective creations, and therefore any evaluation of them must focus on the pictures' psychological content and 'feeling' (Furth, 1988, p. 33). The children may be tempted to evaluate, and sometimes critique, their drawings. Encourage them to name the feelings evoked through the drawings. This will help them become familiar with their own feelings. Jung (Schaverien, 1991, p. 21) understood from his own experience and from observing his patients create drawings, that making pictures was a useful method of getting in touch with the healing aspects of the unconscious.

Overview
    In this lesson, students explore their identity in relation to their home and family relationships.
Recommended age group
    Education providers for ages KS1 and KS2.
Time
    55 minutes approximately.
Preparation
    Hand out a blank paper plate to each child.
    Give the children 15 minutes to draw three images: house, tree and a person on the plate, using crayons. All three images must be on the same side of the plate.
Questions to ask the class
    Ask the class to write their answers to the following questions on the back of their plates:

House – Who lives in the house? Do people visit the house? Is it a happy house? What is the house made of? What goes on inside the house?

Tree – What kind of tree is it? How old is the tree? What season is it? Is the tree alive? Who waters the tree?

Person – Who is the person? How old is the person? How does that person feel? Is the person happy? What does the person like doing?

Interpretation

Collect the plates and reflect on them using this guidance:

The house represents the family relationships and values.

The roof stands for the intellectual and spiritual side.

The walls might be related to the child's character strength.

Doors and windows represent the child's relationship with the outside world and social integration.

The tree is thought to represent the child's deepest unconscious aspects of their personality.

Branches may represent the degree of social connectedness. No branches indicates the child has little contact with others. The trunk is often seen as a representation of inner strength. The tree crown stands for ideas, thoughts and self-concept.

The person is a symbolic representation of the idea of the Self and social interaction. The head symbolises intelligence, communication and imagination. The eyes indicate the perception of the world. The hands represent affectivity and aggressiveness.

Classroom tips

Identify students for whom this topic may be challenging

Children and young people with disabilities or who have experienced abuse, extreme trauma, bereavement or themselves suffer with a mental health condition may find discussions about home and relationships quite challenging. It is important to be aware of these students before teaching this lesson and of any sensitivities or issues that may come up.

Teacher skill: how to build trust and develop a warm, friendly relationship with the child

In a child-centred framework, we create trust and rapport through recognising and supporting the child's agency, respecting their choices and reflecting their feelings back to them. This is the first of Virginia Axline's principles and guides the therapist in all non-directive therapeutic contact with the child. This lets the child know that the therapist has heard them, and we aren't going to use coercive language or tactics to get them to do what we want (if this differs from what they are choosing to do). We will need to be patient and allow the child to choose at all times.

Sometimes this will involve us telling the child about the consequences of their choices. For example, if we are trying to work privately with a child in a room, the child may want the door to remain open (for many reasons: a quick exit is in view, fear of being alone in a room with an adult). A trust-making response would be for us to explain the consequences of this choice to the child rather than either physically closing the door ourselves or insisting that the door remain closed. The decision to close the door needs to be an informed choice that the child makes. If the child becomes angry and aggressive at the idea of the door being closed, reflect their feelings back to them so that they start to recognise and own their own feelings. For example:

Child: I'll smash everything up in here!
You: You're feeling angry now.
Child: I'll smash you up too!
You: You're still feeing angry.

If you responded with a limitation such as 'You can play with all the toys in this room, but you can't smash them up' you are not responding to the child's expressed *feeling*. Don't fall into the trap of reacting to content rather than feeling.

You build trust and rapport by letting the child know you have heard and understood their feelings.

Message box

Protect the child's confidentiality by keeping an empty tissue-sized box on your desk for children to leave their messages in. Cover the box in decorative paper and write 'Message box' clearly so children can read it. Tell them afterwards that if they want to write you a message, to put it into the box at any time of the day and you will read the messages at the end of the day. It's possible that some students will have questions they want to ask you confidentially, not in front of their class mates. This gives them a safe way to do that. Make sure you follow up with any students the following day, and arrange to talk to them privately.

Teacher self-care tip

Building trust can leave you feeling a bit raw, vulnerable. If you feel this way, make sure you do a self-care practice at the end of the day. Wrap yourself up warmly in a cosy blanket, drink a warm drink.

References

Allan, J. (1988). *Inscapes of the Child's World: Jungian Counseling in Schools and Clinics*. Dallas, TX: Spring Publications.

Buck, J.N. (1948). 'The H-T-P', *Journal of Clinical Psychology*, 4, 151–159.

Furth, G.M. (1988). *The Secret World of Drawings: A Jungian Approach to Healing through Art*. Toronto: Inner City Books.

Schaverien, J. (1991). *The Revealing Image: Analytical Art Psychotherapy in Theory and Practice*. London: Routledge.

Chapter 2

Refusal of the Call

Introduction

The hero attempts to refuse the adventure because they are afraid. They may feel unprepared or inadequate, or they may not want to sacrifice what is being asked of them.

Children have been faced with death and loss on a daily basis since March 2020, and this is set to continue for some time. Nothing has prepared them to cope with this challenge. There are some exceptions. Vulnerable children who have experienced loss and threats to their physical and emotional states will have a 'threat awareness', but this will only serve to retraumatise them. In all cases, the loss of freedom and security will make children anxious about accepting this challenge.

The refusal can also be related to other types of change such as moving house. Children resist leaving the familiar behind, their friends and routines, where they play sports, for example. Other types of move can also trigger the refusal such as moving between two homes during a divorce. This can trigger anxiety for children, and lots of anger.

Schools and parents may see behavioural and emotional signs of the children 'acting out' their distress: poor attention span, falling asleep, poor concentration, anger, frustration, sadness, irritability. These are all signs of a child refusing the Call because sometimes the level of change is just too much for them to cope with, and they become dysregulated.

Staying in that dysregulated state is not a happy place, and we don't want a child to remain there. In this place, their options for responding feel limited, and their ability to make cognitive responses unavailable. We need to do two things at the refusal stage:

1. Acknowledge the level of refusal.
2. Enable the child to play out their refusal through a creative medium until they have reached a point of their own resolution.

DOI: 10.4324/9781003182009-4

This will enable them to shift naturally onto the next stage of the hero's journey without being met with punishment or reward. By facilitating this stage with them, you are allowing them to discover their own solution, to work out what they need to accept in order to move on. This stage must not be rushed because if it is, you risk short-circuiting the developmental processing that gives them the capacity to move on. You can't impose a solution. Well you could, but it wouldn't work for very long and, crucially, you would not be acting in the child's best interests, you would be acting against their will, and ignoring the principle of maintaining a deep respect for the child's ability to solve their own problems if given an opportunity to do so (principle 5 of Axline's child-centred framework).

This would set up a situation where you are overpowering the child which is not what we want. We want the child to feel empowered enough to accept the Call, to feel able and ready to say yes. It's important to remember that the refusal stage will take some children longer than others. It's not fair either to generalise and say that all children who have adverse child experiences (ACEs) will automatically struggle with this stage. I have seen some vulnerable children grasp this stage quickly, like a lifeline, as if someone has finally recognised and acknowledged their struggle. So, be mindful not to pre-judge. Test the water by extending the invitation, and go from there with an open mind.

In all cases, the refusal of the Call is the child saying they are not prepared to leave the familiar ground. This is a signal for adults to pay attention and listen. Find out what the refusal is about. Identify the feelings associated with the refusal through this exercise, and help the child to enter this second stage feeling more prepared.

For example, in the film *Star Wars*, Luke Skywalker initially refuses to join Obi-Wan Kenobi on his mission to rescue the princess. It's only when he discovers that his aunt and uncle have been killed by stormtroopers that he changes his mind.

We are going to look at the refusal of the Call in the context of a childhood bereavement.

Case study

EW – who will I cling to if you die?

Edward was 6 years of age when he was referred to me for play therapy by his primary school SENCO in Lincolnshire. He was grieving the death of his Mum who had died six months previously, after a short illness. His father had recently started dating. Edward was angrily resisting the Call to accept both his loss and changed family dynamics.

His Dad's new partner had two young children who Edward had started fighting with. Edward was reeling from his loss and struggling to accept the changes brought about by his Dad's new partner spending more time at their home. New and strange routines were being established with different boundaries, and Edward did not like these changes. Dad maintained a busy work routine and used this to shut down emotionally from Edward. He had less time for Edward, and had started to withdraw from him, not wanting to play football, as he struggled with his own grief. Edward was very confused by his Dad's withdrawal from him, and he had become unsettled and labelled disruptive in his class. He would get up from his desk and wander about the classroom, he was clingy with his teachers, finding it difficult to leave one class and enter the next one. Daily transitions became problematic for Edward. He would cry as he entered the lunch queue if he had to wait what felt like a long time for his lunch. His teachers were struggling to calm him, and he couldn't self-soothe. Dad was 'at his wits end' and found Edward's clinginess unnecessary, and somewhat inexplicable.

Edward refused to accept both his Mum's death and his changed family dynamics, as well as the arrival of a new 'Mum'. This pattern is one which affects one in six children in the UK. The refusal the child is making happens as a reaction to unexpected, unplanned changes, sometimes permanent in the child's life, like a bereavement. When this happens, the child digs in their heels and resists the changes. It is their only way of protesting, if language cannot be used. It's highly unlikely in this primary school age group that a bereaved child would verbally articulate their feelings. Their behaviour will do that for them until this is decoded, which is what needs to happen. Which is where the creative mediums and therapeutic play come in.

Edward and I built a strong and empathic bond, and through the creative media of painting and making crafts, he expressed his feelings of loss and grief. As he learned that it was OK to have his feelings, so he eventually found a level of comfort again within his family.

These weekly sessions took place over an 18-month period. The school was supportive and encouraging of Edward's therapy, and there is no doubt that Edward returned a changed child. Changed because he had been given the gift of space to process his feelings. I held Edward's grief while he struggled with the magnitude of missing his Mum and coming to terms with the reality that he would never see her again. That is a lot for one therapist to hold. Alongside that I was also holding the staff around Edward who were struggling themselves to know how best to support Edward. None of them had received any bereavement and/or therapeutic training. Studies published by the Royal Society of Medicine have revealed many negative outcomes associated with childhood bereavement, e.g. an increased likelihood of substance abuse, greater vulnerability to depression, higher risk of criminal behaviour, school underachievement and lower employment rates. (Ellis, Dowrick and Lloyd-Williams, 2013).

Many interrelated risks and factors mediate or moderate children's experiences; these include factors relating to the child (such as their prior experiences of loss, and coping style), their family and social relationships (including relationship with the person who has died), their wider environment and culture and the circumstances of the death.

There is an 'Edward' in every classroom in this country. Not every school can afford to have this level of therapy, which is why it's crucial that staff are trained in these basic therapeutic play techniques. Not every grieving child can leave the classroom each week.

Theoretical background – understanding bereavement as trauma

Whenever a child or adult is faced with traumatic life events, particularly the loss of a loved one, the ability to survive the emotional and physical pain associated with the event will be influenced by the individual's level of personal resilience (Bunce and Rickards, 2004, p. 1). Factors associated with resilience include secure attachments to significant others, absence of early loss and trauma, high self-esteem, social empathy and an easy temperament. Ethan's attachment style had been disrupted through the loss of his Mum. The family's reduced level of resilience provoked him to adopt attachment-seeking behaviours, which were misunderstood by stressed relatives. Through using the projected play media in the play therapy Toolkit (painting, drawing, clay, sand and music), Edward accessed his 'noticing brain' and gained greater awareness of his thoughts, emotions and sensations.

Separation and loss

Klein says (Bowlby, 1998, p. 93) 'every advance in the process of mourning results in a deepening in the individual's relation to his inner objects'. Edward had a breakthrough while making a picture of his Dad. He sat silently with his head down for a few minutes, and then said: 'I want to make my Daddy happy.' This was something which was missing from his relationship with his Dad, so the fact that Edward felt ready and able to tell me this directly was a sign of his trust in me and the way he was connecting to his feelings. He was expressing his deepest wish. We sat together, bearing what he found so difficult.

What a bereaved child goes through

Furman (1974, p. 163) says that the bereaved child has a threefold task – to cope with the immediate impact of the circumstances, to mourn and to resume and continue his emotional life in harmony with his level of maturity. None of these tasks is completed within a prescribed timeframe. Bereavement has no clock. Depending on internal and external factors, each task may present ongoing difficulties for the bereaved or it may be resolved in such a way as not to impede functioning in later years.

A new pattern emerges

Edward created a series of objects to represent his loss that explored the themes of cutting and imprinting new shapes to create new bonds, all of which symbolised a new stage in his grief process. The new shapes represented his growth in being ready to connect with other nurturing figures in his life.

The first was a sequence of paintings that he created. Before they had dried he cut them out with scissors and imprinted tissue paper onto the wet paintings that covered the painted image. Each stage of this process felt like a huge step emotionally. As he painted the tissue paper, he gave instructions out loud: 'Now we paint this, and now we press it down like this.' There was tremendous energy and strength in the way his body moved during the cutting out and pressing down – he stood at the table (he usually sat) and used his body weight to lean on the table as he pressed down on the tissue paper.

I felt he was creating a new pattern, and felt completely in sync with him as we created these imprints side by side. Each step in the painting process was symbolic of him creating stronger resilience for himself. He chose purple tissue paper which is a colour associated with spirituality and resurrection (Malchiodi, 2007, p. 156). He put his painting and mine into his special box, symbolically including me in this new stage of trust and attachment.

The second object was a bracelet made out of a powder-blue pipe cleaner. He used scissors to cut the pipe cleaner into thirds, and then secured the ends together by twisting them until he had formed a new shape, a circle with twisted knots securing the bracelet together. The knots weren't tight, just loose enough for him to slip the bracelet onto his wrist. Again, I felt the significance of this new shape, the broken, cut circle, similar to the new family he has, with his Mum cut out of the picture through death.

He explored this theme further in the sand. He put a crane into the sand and pulled on the winding chord. When the chord broke, he remained calm and tried to make the crane work without the chord, but gave up trying to make this work when he realised that with the broken chord the attachment of objects to the crane was different and difficult. He noticed this, and I remarked on it. Soon afterwards, he pushed the chord mechanism in with the broken chord, and moved on to drumming and banged the drum loudly. This can happen when a child has connected with their feelings and making a sound with a musical instrument allows them to release the energy that might have been bound up with that emotion. Immediately, the symbolism of the broken chord echoed loudly for me with the broken symbiosis Edward suffered through his mother's death.

After Edward had completed his play therapy, his teacher told me his concentration had improved to the point where he could sit for longer periods of time at his desk and complete his work. This was a huge win for Edward! He was able to settle down at his desk because he had found a settlement within himself. The objects he had created in his sessions, although not a replacement for his mother, were a way for him to project his feelings of loss and begin to find a way to cope with his grief. When the child sees the external objectification of their feeling they feel freer because they are no longer having to contain this feeling themselves.

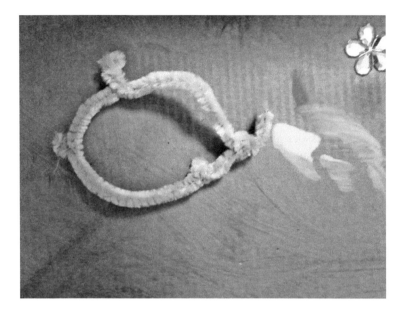

Figure 2.1 Edward's memory bracelet.

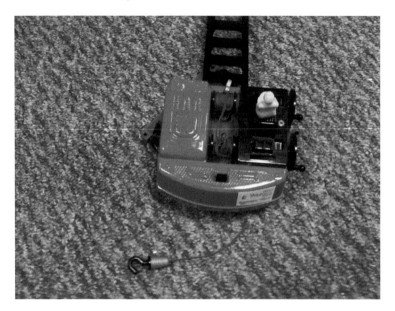

Figure 2.2 Edward's crane showing the broken chord.

Bereavement usually affects a whole family. Any loss resonates with previous losses, which are often reawakened. Where grief is not acknowledged it can damage family relations in a number of ways. The anger of grief may be displaced onto a family member ('scapegoat') who becomes the target of all wrath. This happened in Edward's case where he was blamed for showing his grief. His Dad found this especially difficult to see because he just wanted to move on from his loss and was angry with Edward for not being able to do the same. This was damaging to the parent/child relationship in a number of ways. The trust between father and son became fragile: Edward didn't understand why his Dad was so angry with him and this only made things worse between them. Communication became fraught as his Dad shouted at him to stop being so difficult. Edward didn't understand what he was doing wrong so he became particularly clingy with his Dad, seeking his approval which he rarely got. The one thing Edward's Dad wanted Edward to do was to stop showing him his grief. Edward was expressing his grief in the only way he knew how. Sadly, although the play therapy gave Edward a safe space to express his emotions, his father was unable to cope with his own grief and create a safe space for Edward at home, so the family dynamic of anger continued.

Allowing a family to witness emotional distress in one member can release them to talk about their own feelings (Hospice Education Institute, n.d.).

What do these children need? They need to hear the word 'dead', and they need to hear in a gentle quiet way that their parent is not coming back, although we can understand why they would like that to happen. It was not Daddy or Mummy's choice. A simple explanation of what happened is appropriate, for example: 'Daddy was sick and sometimes the doctors can't fix the problem.' Focusing on words and asking how they feel may be very frustrating for the surviving parent because they may not reach their child in this way. They need to focus on hugs, respecting their child's wish not to be left alone, their child's need to know where their surviving parent is and how they can be found if they leave for a bit. Drawing pictures together, trying to replicate some of what Mummy or Daddy did with and for their child helps. Their child needs to feel cared about and safe.

Lesson plan: making a memory bracelet

Overview

In this lesson, students explore their memories of the person who has died and channel those into creating a bracelet or a box in their memory. This exercise can be used with any type of loss as it helps the child to connect to their memories.

Recommended age group

Education providers for ages KS1 and KS2.

Time

55 minutes approximately.

Preparation

Memory bracelet: Hand out coloured pipe cleaners and raffia.

Memory box: Hand out empty match boxes, sheets of coloured paper, felt tip pens.

Give the children 15 minutes to make their items.

Questions to ask the class

Ask the class to write their answers on a piece of paper. When they have finished, they can either fold it and put it inside their box or keep it separate.

Instructions for making a memory bracelet

These can be made out of raffia or pipe cleaners. The advantage of using raffia is that it has numerous strands which children like to gather together and pull apart until they are happy with the arrangement. The way they play with and organise the raffia into a bracelet usually reflects their level of comfort with their loss. You may need to help them with this and remind them that they are making it as a memory of their loved one. It doesn't have to be perfect, it can be exactly as they want it to be. That means that all the strands don't have to be the same length when they are tied together – all of this is significant in terms of what is says about the child's psyche. You don't need to analyse this, only to note it. The most important aspect about this exercise is to support the child to create the memory bracelet in the way that they want to. When they have finished making the bracelet don't be surprised if they want to give this to you. My advice is to decline this offer and encourage them to keep it by reminding them that they have made a special gift for their loved one. This helps the child to start to come to terms with their loss by owning their feelings associated with that loss.

Instructions for making a memory box

You will need a small box for this exercise, the size of a large matchstick box. Obviously take the matches out before giving it to the child! I keep a collection of these in my practice so I always have them to hand. A couple of sheets of shiny paper, silver and gold, as this is going to be a precious box. Invite the child to choose a sheet and then wrap up the box in the paper and seal it at both ends so that it is covered and secure. A fine-point black pen and some paper. Invite the child to write their special message to their parent on the paper and then cut this out for them and ask them to stick this onto their box.

This is a very powerful exercise to do as the child is literally formulating some of their feelings about their parent. Encourage them to keep this box with them and to hold it when they feel sad or lonely.

Classroom tips

Identify students for whom this topic may be challenging
Children and young people with disabilities or who have experienced abuse, extreme trauma, bereavement or themselves suffer with a mental health condition may find discussions about home and relationships quite challenging. It is important to be aware of these students before teaching this lesson and of any sensitivities or issues that may come up.

Teacher skill – accepting the child exactly as they are

Learning to accept the child exactly as they are sounds easier than it actually is. However, it is a crucial skill to learn not only during this stage of the hero's journey, but throughout. Think of it as the skill that will get you out of a sticky spot (even when your instinct tells you otherwise) and help you to build an empathic relationship with the child. You will recognise a sticky spot because it will prompt you to want to comfort, rescue, fix, change, intervene. Instead, all you have to do is accept.

Let's first look at what acceptance is not.

Acceptance is not:

- Showing impatience, criticism or reproof, either direct or implied.
- Praise.
- Approval.
- Asking questions.
- Making suggestions.
- Starting the play before the child has started in an attempt to 'get things moving'.

These behaviours are all attempts to control the interaction and exchange with the child.

Here is an example of what not showing acceptance looks like (Axline, 1969):

Adult: Did you go to school today?
Child: Yes (followed by silence).
Adult: Did everything go OK today at school?
Child: Yes (more silence).
Adult: You know Jessie, I'm here to support and help you. I wish you would tell me what's upsetting you.
Child: Nothing's upsetting me! (child runs out of room).

You may be familiar with this type of exchange in school. I certainly am. It shows both a desire and frustration on the part of the adult to find out what's upsetting the child. But it's also intrusive and coercive. The child is resentful of the adult's attempt to change their resistance. The child is actively and clearly resisting, and the adult is not accepting that resistance. Instead, the adult is trying to change that resistance into co-operation. This is at the root of all power struggles within families and schools. And, the less accepting you are of what the child is showing you, the more entrenched their resistance to you will become. Think about that. When you see behaviour that is 'at risk' ask yourself what the level of acceptance is in the relationship.

An accepting outcome to consider would be this: if it is obvious that the child does not want to talk, why not be accepting to the extent of letting them sit in silence? And, if silence is what the child wants, be prepared to sit alongside them in that silence until they indicate they are ready to come out of it. Coming out of the silence may not immediately involve talking, so be prepared for your expectations to be confounded. The child may initially move their body out of the silence, change their position in the room or the chair they are sitting on. These are all opportunities for you to reflect back to them that you have noticed their change, and you accept it. This is what starts to build a relationship based on trust, empathy and rapport.

Too often I see schools repeating this cycle with children: 'Tell me what's bothering you', to then conclude there is something mysteriously wrong with the child because they won't explain their feelings. Don't you think they would tell you if they could or wanted to?

Acceptance is:

an attitude of calm, steady, reflective friendliness.

Learn to accept.

References

Axline, M. A. V. M. (1983). *Play Therapy.* New York: Ballantine Books.

Bowlby, J. (1998). *Attachment and Loss, Vol. 3: Loss: Sadness and Depression.* London: Pimlico.

Bunce, M. and Rickards, A. (2004). Working with bereaved children: a guide. The Children's Legal Centre. Available at: www1.essex.ac.uk/armedcon/unit/projects /wwbc_guide/index.html.

Ellis, J., Dowrick, C. and Lloyd-Williams, M. (2013). 'The long-term impact of early parental death: lessons from a narrative study', *Journal of the Royal Society of Medicine*, 106(2), 57–67.

Furman, E. (1974). *A Child's Parent Dies: Studies in Childhood Bereavement.* New Haven, CT: Yale University Press.

Hospice Education Institute (n.d.). 'Family therapy'. Available at: https://www. hospiceuk.org/what-we-offer/;publications. Accessed 17 May 2022.

Malchiodi, C.A. (2007). *The Art Therapy Sourcebook.* New York: McGraw-Hill.

Chapter 3

Meeting the mentor

Introduction

The mentor is one of the archetypes drawn from the depth psychology of Carl Jung and the mythic studies of Joseph Campbell. Here, we are looking at the mentor as Christopher Vogler does in his book, *The Writer's Journey: Mythic Structure for Writers* (2020). All three of these 'modern' men help us to understand the mentor's role in humanity, in the myths that guide our lives, including religions, and in our storytelling, which is what we will focus on here.

The mentor

The mentor is the wise old man or woman every hero meets fairly early in the most satisfying stories. The role is one of the most recognisable symbols in literature. Think Dumbledore from *Harry Potter*, Q from the James Bond series, Gandalf from *Lord of the Rings*, Yoda from *Star Trek*, Merlin from *King Arthur and the Knights of the Round Table*, Alfred from *Batman*, the list is very long. Even Mary Poppins is a mentor. How many others can you think of?

The mentor represents the bond between parent and child, teacher and student, doctor and patient, God and man. The function of the mentor is to prepare the hero to face the unknown, to accept the adventure. Athena, the goddess of wisdom, is the full, undiluted energy of the mentor archetype, according to Vogler.

Meeting with the mentor

In most hero's journey stories, the hero is first seen in the *ordinary world* when they receive a *call to adventure*. Our hero generally refuses that call initially, either afraid of what will happen or satisfied with life as it is. And then someone like Gandalf appears to change the hero's mind, and to bestow gifts and gadgets. This is the 'meeting with the mentor'.

The mentor gives the hero the supplies, knowledge and confidence required to overcome their fear and face the adventure. Bear in mind that the mentor doesn't have to be a person. The job can be accomplished by a map or experience from a previous adventure.

In *The Wizard of Oz*, Dorothy meets a series of mentors: Professor Marvel, Glinda the Good Witch, Scarecrow, Tin Man, the Cowardly Lion and the Wizard himself.

Think about why the hero's relationship with the mentor or mentors is important to the story. One reason is usually that readers can relate to the experience. They enjoy being a part of an emotional relationship between hero and mentor.

Who are the mentors in your story? Are they obvious or subtle? Has the author done a good job of turning the archetype on its head in a surprising way? Or is the mentor a stereotypical fairy godmother or white-bearded wizard? Some authors will use the reader's expectations of such a mentor to surprise them with a completely different kind of mentor.

Watch for mentors when a story seems stuck. Mentors are the ones who provide aid, advice or magical equipment when all appears doomed. They reflect the reality that we all have to learn life's lessons from someone or something.

The hero encounters someone who can give them advice and ready them for the journey ahead. Acting as a mentor, this person imparts wisdom, which may then change the hero's mind.

In traditional storytelling, the mentor imparts wisdom to the hero, which can make the hero sound passive. In reality, and particularly in the context of storytelling where 'active engagement' is required, this mentor doesn't just impart wisdom, they learn how to interact and engage with the child so that the child learns to trust and discover their own wisdom as well. Principles such as 'unconditional positive regard' (Carl Rogers) mean that a therapeutic alliance characterised by a deep respect and genuine acceptance will nurture the child's capacity for healing and self-determination. It means caring for the child as a separate person, with permission to have their own feelings, their own experiences (Kirschenbaum and Henderson, 1990, p. 225).

When the mentor appears, the hero needs to be ready to meet the challenge. In mythical stories, the mentor shows up already full of wisdom, like Obi-Wan Kenobi, whereas in reality, wisdom is a quality that must be learned. The skills required by the mentor to be ready to meet the child and to be fully engaged are described in 'Teacher skills' at the end of each chapter.

As Dennis McCarthy says:

> What gets depicted needs to be tolerated by us and not 'made nice' or interpreted. What the story or imagery means to the child is felt by her already in its very depicting. Our active witnessing it is a crucial piece of both its appearance and its resolution. And our knowing that it has meaning is even more important than knowing what that meaning is.
>
> (McCarthy, 2012, p. 29)

It will be through the quality of the relational bond between adult and child that the child learns the strength of their own wisdom. This message is at the heart of child-centred play therapy.

What I'm seeking to do here is advocate for a version of the hero's journey that blends the child-centred principles of play therapy into the storytelling framework.

The mentor could be a teacher or therapist, someone the child trusts. It is through the relationship that the child builds confidence to learn and trust their own judgement, decisions and intuitions. This relationship needs to be one where the child can experiment, unpack their emotional backpack, get messy and feel safe. There may be fall outs, walk outs, meltdowns by the child in the course of this relationship. During these times, the mentor needs to remain steady and calm, hold the boundaries for the child to rail within and against. The message here is, 'everything you bring and show me is OK, I'm not leaving you'. If the mentor is a therapist, they will be trained to hold the child's process.

I fill the role of mentor in the following case study. The play therapy kit provides the 'gifts and gadgets', and you see our relationship form, develop and change throughout the child's weekly sessions. You see the impact this has on me and on the child and how a secure attachment makes space for the push and pull rather than trying to control or shut this down. Ultimately the child realises that the question she is asking – How do I know I can trust you? – has its roots in being able to trust herself, her judgements, decisions and feelings. This is the root of real wisdom. It emerges slowly from within the Self. The mentor, in this case me in the role of therapist, is there to meet the child and partner with them through this stage of their hero's journey until they have learnt all they need to, and are ready to move onto the next stage, taking those lessons with them.

Case study

J - How do I know I can trust you?

Source of referral

This case presents a 7-year-old girl called Jane with a pre-strengths and difficulties questionnaire (SDQ) score of 21, in Year 3 at the Malcolm Sargent Primary School in Lincolnshire. I saw Jane for twelve individual play therapy sessions, after which her SDQ reduced to thirteen. Jane initially presented as uncontained with skittish, erratic movement. She developed into a child who found her voice, developed containment strategies and became engaged with self-directing and sharing her play.

The SENCO referral noted Jane's extremely defiant and complex behaviour. She could show limited remorse and continued to push and test 'ultimate consequence' boundaries. The cause of her behaviour was listed as unknown, but the SENCO's concern was that Jane displayed attachment difficulties, although her home life seemed stable. Jane was therefore a bit of a puzzle.

Hoped for outcomes

I explained that the use of reflections during play therapy with repetitive calming messages would release GABA – anti-anxiety chemicals which when released into the brain modify any trauma (*Play for Life Journal*, 2007, pp. 2–3).

It was hoped that Jane would show:

- A greater understanding of her behaviours.
- An awareness of consequences.
- Be more settled in class, less defiant.
- Show remorse when she was in the wrong.

Play Therapy Dimensions Model

The sessions were non-directed, with a relatively low level of consciousness, as Jane preferred to play in a symbolic and metaphorical manner, which was appropriate given her insecure attachment style. There were occasions when I made comments that directly linked Jane's play themes to known elements of Jane's experiences, but the majority of my interpretations were reflective. The play was responsive and non-intrusive, where Jane initiated and directed her play (Quadrant 3), and I joined in her play at her invitation and direction.

There were some occasions when I moved into the conscious surface of Quadrant 2 and asked Jane some open questions, and towards the end of each session I brought Jane back into the conscious surface before she returned to her class. Strong archetypal themes appeared combined with transference and counter-transference (Yasenik, 2012).

Parental interview

Mr and Mrs H consented to the play therapy sessions and completed the pre-SDQ. Both parents worked full-time in the prison service, and Jane was frequently collected by her grandparents from her after-school club. Mrs H's work took her away from home mid-week. They had a younger daughter, E, aged 5. Both children lived with both their parents. English was the spoken language at home. The parents admitted their work schedules did not allow them much time for playing together as a family, but believed that this was balanced out by being able to provide the children with day-out treats and holidays. Jane told me and her teaching assistant (TA) that she didn't want her Mummy to work so that she could be with her.

Her parents described Jane's behaviour as being 'up and down', with their main concern being her defiance of boundaries and angry outbursts in response to hearing 'No'. They said her tantrums started at 15 months, the same time that she suffered a head injury from which she physically recovered. No reference was made to the potential emotional or neurological impact this trauma may have had on Jane. They described Jane as playing well with her extended family, and being loving towards them both. I felt quite tense with both parents and wondered whether they found it difficult to switch off at home from their respective work routines, and how strict they were with disciplining Jane. They struggled to understand why Jane was more difficult to handle than her sister, and I sensed Mrs H's increasing frustration about being unable to understand and control Jane.

Johnson (2008, p. 28) argues that 'any emotional impact we experience is inside us', which is the result of that emotion being projected onto us. Throughout this case, a key part of my learning in supervision was to name the process of my projections, and to ask questions about why I had such strong feelings when I looked at Jane. As Johnson (2008, p. 29) says, this was the beginning of me becoming more conscious, and a key to establishing empathy with Jane.

Talking about the narcissistic disturbance of the mother, Miller (1990, p. 52) argues that when the mother cannot take care of her own narcissistic needs and love her child in the way that the child needs to be loved, continuity and constancy are missing from this love.

Miller concludes by saying that what is missing is the 'framework within which the child could experience his feelings and his emotions'. I wondered if this framework was missing, and had had a negative impact on Jane's ability to form healthy self-esteem.

Embodiment – Projection – Role

According to Dr Sue Jennings (1999, p. 14), competence in embodiment-projection-role (EPR) is essential for a child's maturation. EPR is a developmental paradigm which charts the progression of dramatic play from birth to 7 years through three stages: embodiment stage (sensory and physical); projection stage (engagement with people and things outside the child's physical world); and role stage (dramatising their play through various roles). The early attachment between mother and infant has a dramatic component through playfulness and 'role-reversal'. Assessing Jane using this model for dramatic play, I observed her pass through all three stages, spending most of her sessions playing in the projective stage through paint, sand, clay, music and soft toys. Initially her spatial awareness was poor, she knocked paint bottles over by failing to judge the proximity of bottles in front of her, unaware of where her arms and hands were in relation to items on the table. This did improve. During the role stage, she developed hide-and-seek games which she directed, and took on the role of being the baby, while I became the mother who read bedtime stories to her.

Supervision

I experienced strong transference and counter-transference, which I processed during supervision. I wanted to rescue Jane, make her feel secure, and these anxieties brought me face-to-face with my own archetypal shadow, something I had recognised during my diploma sandtrays. Jung (1990, p. 20) describes the shadow as the 'apprentice-piece' in a person's development. It represents the personal unconscious as a whole, and aspects of a person's dark side, which aren't consciously acknowledged. I learnt to point out certain risks to Jane, and ask her what she wanted to do about them, which enabled Jane to make her own decisions. Asking her an open question often led us into a discussion about her choices.

Through this discussion Jane became more aware of being able to rescue herself, which, in turn, reduced my anxiety. Instead of knocking the paint bottle over, Jane moved it to a safe place. During this open discussion and exploration, we had shifted into a more conscious state recognised as Quadrant 2 in the Play Therapy Dimensions Model (PTDM).

Preliminary session: establishing a contract

Halprin (2003, p. 146) argues that our bodies express our emotions through posture and gesture, in the ways we move when we are stuck, and the quality of our longing or our joy.

My first impression was that Jane struggled to contain her frenetic energy within her physical body. She darted around the room looking at the toys. Over time I learnt that this movement was a reflection of her anxiety, just as being able to lie down on the blanket during later sessions was a reflection of her having reached a more relaxed state. Her posture was initially a little stooped, but over the course of her sessions her spine straightened and she stood taller, a reflection perhaps of having discovered a stronger sense of Self, and a secure base. During her preliminary session she managed to sit at the painting table while I explained the rules. She decorated her special box on the outside, and answered the SDQ which scored 9. The early transference made me feel alarmed, tense, on the alert, imprisoned during the session.

My early assessment of Jane's issues were an insecure and ambivalent attachment to her mother, which had resulted in an insecure base and bond. This left Jane feeling insecure about herself and how to feel safe, and boundaried with other people.

Core Self

Throughout this case I used the HTP drawing tool to assess Jane's unconscious difficulties. According to John Buck (Wikipedia, 2012), the house symbolises the core Self. The houses in Jane's drawings looked empty, lopsided and fragile. I felt sad and lost reflecting on these drawings. The person symbolises the ego. The people in Jane's drawings were not well defined and had missing limbs. The tree symbolises rootedness and security. Janes trees had no roots.

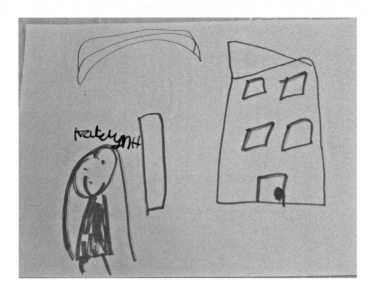

Figure 3.1 HTP drawing 1. A feeling of disconnection is transmitted in this drawing in the way the house, tree and person don't link up.

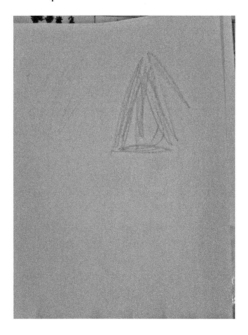

Figure 3.2 HTP drawing 2. An overwhelming feeling of chaos in this drawing. The blue in the top (attic) part of the house might refer to triggered memories and feelings stirred up during the session.

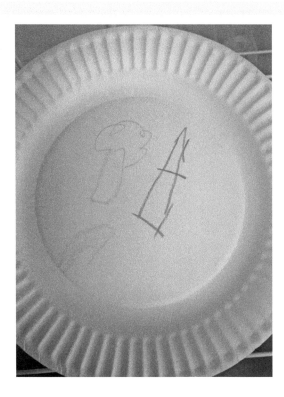

Figure 3.3 This drawing shows an indistinctive house, tree and person. The red triangular shape is slightly lopsided and feels awkward, with no inner sign of detail or, perhaps, life. The tree has no roots and the person appears to be missing.

Her process of activating individuation started with her painted faces and mandala paintings, what Jung (1990, p. 304) refers to as 'the psychological expression of the totality of the self'. Moving through the alchemical mixing of sand and water, she was able to strengthen her core Self sufficiently to be able to contain herself and work within the boundaries of the classroom, a place she was temporarily excluded from during her play therapy.

Testing boundaries

Whitfield (1993, p. 50) argues that if a child's family of origin and environment are unhealthy, through the process of teaching and modelling, the child will learn and develop an unhealthy sense of Self and unhealthy boundaries. I wondered if the rigidity of the parental boundaries made it hard for Jane to explore, which made her push against them.

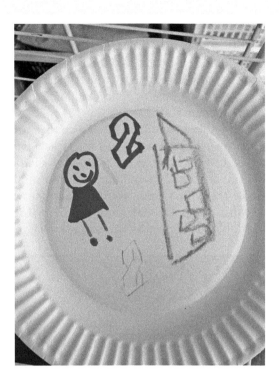

Figure 3.4 Purple image, which represents the house, feels like
chaos remains in the house, symbolised by the windows
being situated on top of each other. It looks uncomfortable without much space for movement or safety.
Person: a girl, with hair and a smile, but her arms are
missing suggesting a lack of agency. The most distinctive
person Jane drew.

Jane tested all the room boundaries I set up: spilling water on the floor
while pouring water into teapots, removing the glitter lids, spilling sand
outside the sandtray and spilling paint over the edges of all five paint pots
following a lot of swirling and stirring. This showed me how she was emotionally spilling out, and struggling to find a secure, safe place to hold her
Self, relying on me to pull her back inside the boundaries. In supervision
I became aware of how her push/pull behaviour was a reflection of her
ambivalent, insecure attachment. I deepened my awareness of how she
wanted the freedom that came with removing the glitter pot lid altogether,
and wondered about this new opening she had created, and how liberating
that felt for her, given the closed door in her HTP drawing. Recognising the
significance of this wider opening, I gave Jane a foil tray which she used to
mix sand, water and glitter. This marked a new stage in her processing.

Activating the process of individuation through mandalas

Kellogg (APAC, 2014) argues that the close alignment of ego and Self is revealed when young children create mandala drawings. Their mandalas reflect the fact that the ego is developing within the matrix of the Self.

Using Kellogg's assessment, Jane painted mandalas in stages 2 (Bliss), 4 (Target) and 12 (Transcendental Ecstasy).

During the painting of these mandalas, I felt a connection between Jane's swirling energy and the vibrant, mandala targets she painted, while the edges of the paper plates represented the boundary she contained herself within. Jane predominantly used the colour red, and mixed this with the colour white to make the colour pink. By this stage she was managing to contain her paint within the pots. Malchiodi (2007, p. 158) associates the colour red with birth, blood, fire, emotion, warmth, love, passion, wounds,

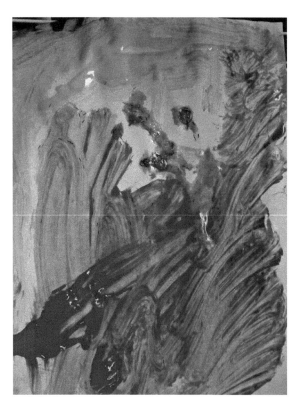

Figure 3.5 First face: two red circles resemble eyes. The left eye is less distinct than the right eye and a nose stuck together with glitter glue. The beginning of identity and Jane recognising her Self.

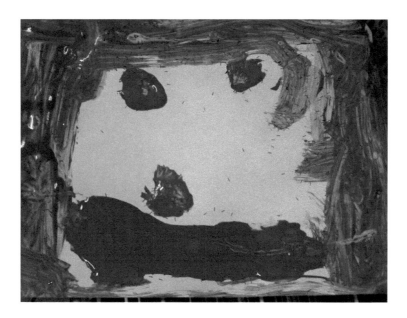

Figure 3.6 More distinctive red dotted eyes, marks perhaps of Jane
claiming this part of her 'seeing' Self. A large red mouth
appears, symbolising Jane's emerging voice.

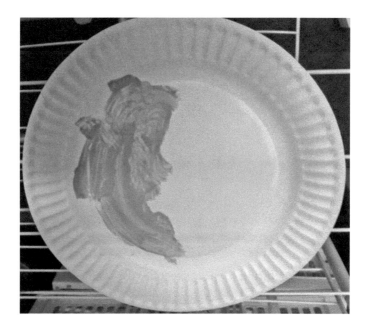

Figure 3.7 Mandala 1.

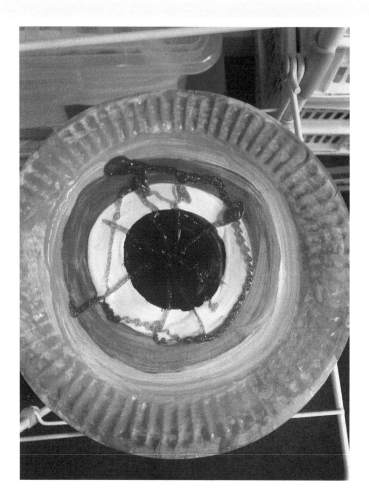

Figure 3.8 Mandala 2.

anger, heat and life. Within Jane's swirling paint mixing and paintings, I felt the heat and anger surfacing which I was able to reflect back to her. There was a new purposeful sound to her voice, as she stated clearly what she was doing, and wanted me to do, directing me to take part in her colour mixing process. I felt we were like a couple of magicians mixing a special potion.

Regressing to feel nurtured

Jane reached a point during session 8 where she wanted to be covered up with the blanket and drink from the baby bottle, while I read her a story. I turned the light off, which she wanted me to do, and we sat together cosily on the blue blanket. She drew nearer to me while drinking, and I felt a strong attachment forming. Afterwards she lay down on the blue blanket

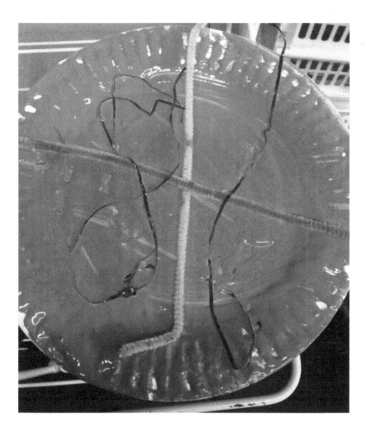

Figure 3.9 Mandala 3.

and hugged a teddy bear, telling him how much she loved him. Then she asked me to hide the marbles and coloured stones for her to find. Afterwards I was aware of the transference between us because I felt hungry, and ate some food. I felt Jane had necessarily regressed to being a younger child in order to receive the nurturing she had perhaps missed out on within her primary attachment relationships.

Parental feedback

I used supervision to explore how I could give uncharged parental feedback. The source of my charge was a feeling of judgement towards Jane's parents which tapped directly into my unconscious fear of the Ruler archetype, who both drew and repelled my need to control chaos (Pearson, 1991). This counter-transference made me afraid of being told off. We decided on an indirect approach, which avoided shaming Jane's parents and provoking their need to control situations. Bearing in mind Jane's hugging of the teddy, I said how difficult it might be for Jane to ask them for cuddles, and

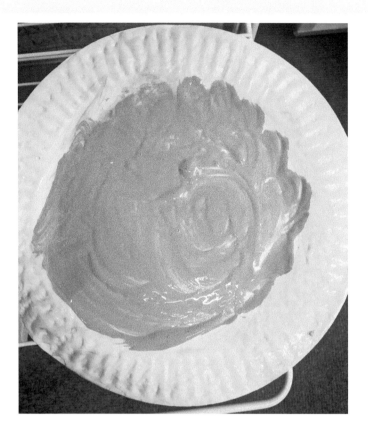

Figure 3.10 Mandala 4.

encouraged them to cuddle her. Again this mirrored my own fear of being rejected, and was a painful awareness to reach during these sessions.

Hearing a cry for help

I didn't see Jane for several weeks during her school exclusion. I was aware of not reacting to this situation so that I could accept whatever Jane showed me when she returned to her sessions. Through clay making Jane learnt to stay away from the heat. She did this by cutting up clay into small pieces, placing them onto four picnic plates, and positioning the plates in front of the fan heater to cook, while she watched the clay soften! I reminded her to move herself and her plate further away from the heater. This felt like a metaphor for the way she got too close to the heat at school. She pulled herself and her plate away from the heater, and showed me how soft the clay was. We examined and touched this plasticine. I wondered if this softened clay was symbolic of Jane's soft centre, a centre she could feel when she was caught up in the fiery energy and heat of defiance, discipline and confrontation, something I could relate to.

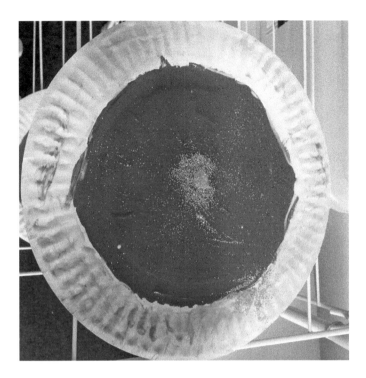

Figure 3.11 **Mandala 5.**

Setting my boundaries

Upon her return to school, Jane was assigned a TA, and a Team Around the Child (TAC) meeting was set up. I resisted my first instinct to offer to attend these meetings, and took this into supervision where I addressed my need to fix, rescue and hold emotional baggage that didn't belong to me. Instead I wrote a mid-review report for the SENCO which was welcomed. This allowed me to remain contained, and more available to hold and process with Jane.

The beginning of transformation

Jung (1958) believed that alchemy was a symbolic representation of the individual's individuation (separation) process, and that these individual psychic processes were genetically encoded.

When Jane started mixing sand, water and glitter glue to create a new substance, I felt she was in a transformational process (Bradway and McCoard, 2010). Once this transformation had taken place, she played with the new substance and repeated the process. She began using picnic cups and teapots to mix and contain sand and water, and to create a new substance. She directed me to take part in this process, and we poured sand from the sandtray into a foil tray, then into individual cups and finally into small glasses.

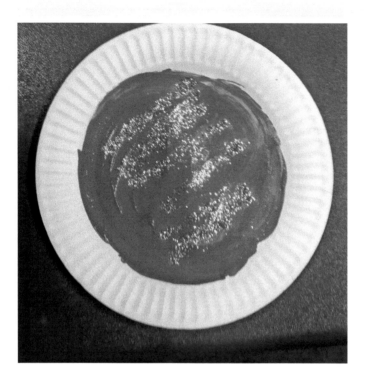

Figure 3.12 **Mandala 6.**

The pouring of sand into the water along with stirring became a joint weekly activity. She was careful to lay out a plastic tablecloth over the carpet, and managed the transition of water from bowl into cup well. The final mixture was poured by Jane into the plastic baby bottle, before squeezing the teet to expel the water into the glasses, from which we then pretended to drink. I felt I was being fed like a baby, and could see and feel that the play and relationship was allowing Jane to feed herself.

The dissolution of the sand into the water created other changes in Jane's play. There was no more banging the drum and clashing of the Tibetan bells. Some of her opposing energies had harmonised as she had started her individuation process.

Towards the end of her sessions, her TA reported that Jane's class behaviour had improved, and she had started to share with her classmates, which was a huge improvement. Previously she had struggled with this aspect of peer behaviour.

Celebrations

We celebrated the ending with a chocolate picnic which Jane devoured! She painted her final mandala before repeating the sand process again. I felt

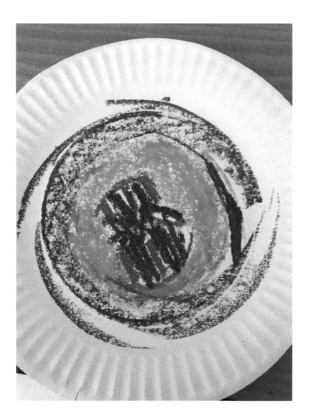

Figure 3.13 Final mandala 7.

happy, and she kept smiling at me with lots of direct eye contact. Her body movements had slowed down, and she was now more measured and controlled, no jerks. She listened when I told her to step off the plastic floor covering so that I could pull out the wrinkles so that she would not slip, all to keep her safe. Before we left the room for the final time, Jane carefully gathered up her painting folder and box, and said goodbye to me and all the toys.

Aims achieved

From the school's point of view, Jane had made good progress in terms of achieving their hoped for outcomes. She understood the consequences of her behaviour, and responded well to boundary setting rather than traffic light behaviour. She was able to work alone without her TA most of the time, but still wanted some reassurance of help when required.

Parent end review

Both parents reported that Jane was calmer, seemed happier, more tolerant and her school work had improved. She was having fewer tantrums, and beginning to show remorse if she was in the wrong. She was opening up to them a little before bedtime, which was a big change. There was a 50% improvement in being able to respect boundaries, but they saw no real improvement in her concentration. Her parents had started saying that police were 'good people', and Jane had responded to that change in attitude. However, they were still concerned about Jane's extreme emotional reaction when something happened beyond her control, and noticed that she had started picking her scabs again and twiddling her hair in response to feeling anxious. The school, together with her parents, had referred Jane to a paediatrician regarding attention deficit hyperactivity disorder (ADHD). They agreed to try and delay the use of Ritalin, and as a family had agreed to become involved in a Nottingham University ADHD test.

I felt satisfied that Jane could now stand up for herself without alienating people, and pushing them away. Through her play and our relationship she had experienced a more secure form of attachment, and learned to trust me and herself.

Theoretical background – understanding attachment as a grief print

When a child reaches this stage in their journey, their attachment style will become apparent. The way a child grieves their losses will to some extent be determined by their attachment style. Research completed by Dr Colin Murray Parkes shows us that the attachment style and vulnerability that is evident in childhood continues into adult life and may have an impact on the way individuals react to losses such as bereavements in adult life. How our attachments develop in childhood can influence how far we can trust ourselves and others in our life. Crucially, our attachment style may affect our ability to form coping strategies when an important close relationship is lost. This loss can be felt through distance as well as through death. As we see in this case study, the parents were felt by the child to be emotionally distant as well as physically absent. She experienced this absence as a loss of closeness and connection, and all that this implied: reliability and constancy. So whenever a loss is felt, the child will defer to their attachment style (grief print) to cope.

Dr Parkes studied a sample of 278 individuals referred to him by a general physician, often with loss-related problems. His work discusses attachment styles and describes them as being:

Secure: Those whose parents provided security grow up trusting themselves and others, which enables them to be able to tolerate separations without suffering high anxiety. Although they may struggle with unexpected losses, they may cope well with the changes the losses bring and use them to discover new meaning.

Anxious/Ambivalent: Those whose parents were anxious, overprotective and/or insensitive to meeting their child's need for independence tend to grow up being anxious, with low self-confidence and with a tendency to cling to their parents. They tend to struggle with separating from their parents, and their relationships in adult life may contain a lot of conflict. After a bereavement their anxiety dominates their behavior and they may cling to those trying to support them. Children with this attachment style may show a tendency to form dependent relationships which teachers need to be aware of.

Avoidant: Those whose parents were intolerant of intimacy and expressing emotion learn to be inhibited from emotional displays and to be independent from an early age. They may become intolerant of intimacy which can complicate their adult relationships. Following bereavement, they tend to be inhibited in their grief which may then show up in distorted ways. They are often hard on themselves for their inability to express their feelings and may respond positively to a relationship which allows them to be expressive.

Disorganised: Those whose parents' emotional needs made it impossible for them to respond consistently to their child's needs may grow up feeling helpless about their own needs and distrusting themselves and others. Bereavement can make them panic and also give them a chance to discover that not everyone will let them down.

Teachers can provide children with the secure base that makes them feel safe enough to take on their challenges. One way they can do this is by offering the children the tool of creating a mandala, which will help them to meet their 'inner mentor' and activate their inner wisdom. Through doing this, and being safely held by the teacher in the relationship, they will learn to trust themselves.

Lesson plan: activating the process of individuation

Mandalas

Mandala is Sanskrit for 'circle' and also for 'completion'. It has been a symbol of wholeness and connection to Spirit in all cultural developments. Drawing or colouring a mandala can be meditative. As you focus your attention on colouring in the patterns of the mandala, your body relaxes, your thoughts slow down, the mind becomes quiet and you may find yourself entering a spiritual space. Mandalas are found in the Early Christian Celtic Cross, prayer circles, Hindu sand mandalas, Native American dream catchers and medicine wheels, Stonehenge, the human cell and the campfire.

The nature of drawing a mandala is therapeutic and symbolic. The shapes and colours you choose will be a reflection of your inner Self at the time of creation. Psychoanalyst Carl Jung described the mandala as a graphical representation of the centre, the unconscious Self. It can appear in dreams and visions or it can be created as a work of art.

Overview

When mandalas are used in therapy, the therapist uses a mandala created by the client as a representation of their current feelings and emotions. The technique of creating a mandala can be self-calming and self-centring.

This tool will enable children to express their feelings wherever they are in their journey.

Recommended age group
    Education providers for ages KS1 and KS2.
Time
    55 minutes approximately.
Preparation
    Read the story 'Eric and the Frog' out loud to the class.

Hand out a circle drawn on a piece of paper to each child and provide some coloured crayons. Ask them to create their mandala to 'show how you feel today' in response to the story.

    Give them 15 minutes to make their mandala.

    Teaching children about mandalas can give them a tool to use at home for relaxation and self-soothing. Some children may enjoy keeping a 'mandala journal' in which they create a different mandala every day as a way of increasing mindfulness and self-awareness.

Classroom tips

Identify students for whom this topic may be challenging

Children and young people with disabilities or who have experienced abuse, extreme trauma, bereavement or themselves suffer with a mental health condition may find discussions around home and relationships quite challenging. It is important to be aware of these students before teaching this lesson and of any sensitivities or issues that may come up.

Eric and the Frog

Eric lived with his Mum and Dad near the woods. Every day before and after school Eric ran outside and played in the woods. Every day he found new treasure, a stone to add to his collection, a feather to build a nest with. There was a never ending supply of rocks and wood that Eric could make things out of. One morning Eric found something very different in the woods … something he had never seen before. Eric's eyebrows shot up and his heart started racing. It was a bullfrog! Very green and very large lying on his side making a sound that reminded Eric of his sister choking on her food.

    Eric ran over to the frog thinking it might be dead but he saw that the frog's eyes were slowly blinking and he realised he was still alive. Eric wondered what to do – he didn't want to be late for school but he couldn't just leave this poor frog fighting to breathe, so he ran back to his house to call his Mum.

    'Mum, come quick, I've found a frog in the woods and I think he needs help. Bring water!', Eric shouted. He filled a small plant pot with water from the garden hose and walked as quickly as he could back to the woods. He hoped the frog was still alive, he hoped he wasn't too late.

    Meanwhile his Mum, looking out the window, saw Eric filling the pot with water and called his Dad. His Dad called his sister, who brought a wet towel and, pretty soon, they were all gathered together in the woods looking at the frog with Eric.

Eric knelt down next to the frog and quietly dabbed him with water from his pot. The frog's choking sounds eased off and he stopped blinking his eyes. Eric looked at his Dad. 'Don't frogs live in ponds?', he said. His Dad nodded. 'Hold on, frog', said Eric. 'We are going to find you a pond and you will be home soon.' The frog let out a little sigh.

Then everyone worked together to find the pond in the woods. Eric's sister found it first: 'It's over here', she shouted. Eric and his Mum carefully lifted the frog onto a wet towel and carried him to the pond. Eric was holding his breath, willing the frog to stay alive. They released the frog into the water and saw the life come back into him. His legs quivered and he wriggled his body as he began to swim in the water.

Eric stood up and let out a loud cheer: 'Yay, we did it!'

The next day, Eric returned to the pond to check on his frog. He looked at all sides of the pond and eventually sat down and stared at the water watching it for any ripples. Finally his Mum came to find him, and put her arm around him. She said, 'I am really proud of you, Eric.' Then they slowly walked back to the house together.

(Seyderhelm, 2020)

Teacher skill – actively witnessing the emergence of something new

The key elements of active witnessing are listening and patience. In order to be patient, it is helpful to remember Nancy Levin's advice to honour the space between 'no longer and not yet'.

Let's look at these elements more closely through an example of another case study.

Hayden, a client, no longer wanted to take part in school sports. He would get into fights with his team mates which would lead to him being asked to withdraw from the game and sit on the sidelines. Sitting there, he brooded not only on his exclusion from the game, but also on his anger at not feeling part of the team. He didn't know why, and neither did I. When he started play therapy he was in the space between 'no longer and not yet'. Offering him strategies to try at this point would have amounted to me rescuing him and interfered with his process of learning about himself. He needed to understand which part of him was not being fully heard and witnessed. So during this 'no longer and yet' stage, we began the session each week by playing cards, a game Hayden indicated he wanted to play with me. This was the start of his beginning to know. Could he trust me? Was I a worthy competitor (a quality that was important to Hayden)? Would I judge him when he cheated? Would I tell him to stop expressing himself loudly when he won? Over time, as I listened and reflected back to him his anger and frustration at losing, he realised that I wasn't judging him, I was accepting him, and he started to relax and to accept himself.

As Dennis McCarthy says, even though the emotions exposed in play therapy are quite often expressed via symbol or metaphor, the emotions are still there, benefiting from us witnessing them. It is our presence in the play experience that makes it therapeutic. As witness we serve as both mirror and other which is a powerful duo and that is what facilitates the potential emergence of something new.

When you are faced with a child who is at this stage, be the mentor and guide that they need simply by actively witnessing what they are expressing. Get out of your own way – remember, this is not about you – see the story, sense its importance and allow yourself to be moved by it together with the child. Be simultaneously in the story-making with the child and also separate enough from it to observe, witness and record it. As McCarthy says, this serves as both a link to the present and also as an instigator of the deeper feelings that are allowed to surface through the play.

Be ready to step in when needed, to engage in the child's play playfully, accepting the dichotomy of the serious and the banal. What you are doing is both emphatically accepting the complex and contradictory emotions and impulses in the child and also not attempting to resolve them. This is both essential and very hard, the foundation of being patient while they unpack their feelings for you. This is the essence of you learning to decode, something we will look at next.

References

Academy of Play and Child Psychotherapy (APAC) (2014). Diploma in *Play Therapy Course*. Uckfield, East Sussex: APAC.

Bradway, K. and McCoard, B. (2010). *Sandplay – Silent Workshop of the Psyche*. London: Routledge.

Halprin, D. (2003). *The Expressive Body in Life, Art and Therapy: Working with Movement, Metaphor and Meaning*. London: Jessica Kingsley Publishers.

Jennings, S. (1999). *Introduction to Developmental Play Therapy*. London:. Jessica Kingsley Publishers.

Johnson, R.A. (2008). *Inner Gold. Understanding Psychological Projection*. Ashville, NC: Koa Books.

Jung, C.J. (1958). *Psyche and Symbol*. New York: Doubleday.

Jung, C.J. (1990). *The Archetypes and the Collective Unconscious*. London: Routledge.

Kirschenbaum, H. and Henderson, V.L. (eds) (1990). *The Carl Rogers Reader. Reflections from the Lifetime Work of America's Preeminent Psychologist*. London: Constable.

Malchiodi, C.A. (2007). *The Art Therapy Sourcebook*. New York: McGraw-Hill. maricreativeresources.com.

McCarthy, D. (2012). *A Manual of Dynamic Play Therapy: Helping Things Fall Apart, the Paradox of Play*. London: Jessica Kingsley Publishers.

Miller, A. (1990). *The Drama of Being a Child*. London: Virago.

Pearson, C.S. (1991). *Awakening the Heroes Within*. New York, HarperCollins.

Play Therapy UK and Play Therapy International (PTUK and PTI) (2007). *Play for Life, The Journal of Play Therapy International and its Affiliates*. Uckfield, East Sussex, PTUK.

Seyderhelm, A. (2020). *Helping Children Cope with Loss and Change: A Guide for Professional and Parents.* Oxford: Routledge.

Vogler, C. (2020). *The Writer's Journey: Mythic Structure for Writers.* Studio City, CA: Michael Wiese Productions.

Whitfield, C.L. (1993). *Boundaries and Relationships: Knowing, Protecting, and Enjoying the Self.* Florida: Health Communications Inc.

Wikipedia, (2012). *House Tree Person Test* (Online). Available at: https://en.wikipedia.org/wiki/House-Tree-Person_test. Accessed 17 August 2015.

Yasenik, L. (2012). *Play Therapy Dimensions Model: A Decision-Making Guide for Integrative Play Therapists.* London: Jessica Kingsley Publishers.

Chapter 4

Crossing the first threshold

Introduction

The hero leaves his ordinary world for the first time, and crosses the threshold into adventure. This step may seem almost inevitable, but it also represents a choice the hero is making. It is a door through which the hero must pass for the story to really begin.

When the child is ready to cross the threshold it generally means that they have begun the process of identifying themselves through a metaphor which has appeared in either a story or their play. This is a momentous stage for them to have reached, perhaps for the first time, the act of feeling recognised.

Metaphor gives children a 'safe distance' from which to identify with characters going through similar struggles. The character's journey enables them to express their feelings, and ultimately resolve their inner and outer conflicts.

Some of the threats children are facing will evoke big feelings and they can find safety in story characters.

It is easier for adults to start conversations with children about their feelings through story characters, and learn what the children need and how to help them.

For example, in *The Lord of the Rings*, Frodo and Sam literally cross the threshold between the world they've known, The Shire, to a world they are unfamiliar with – beyond The Shire. In the 1986 coming-of-age film *Stand by Me*, the boys walk onto the train tracks leading away from their hometown of Castle Rock – and it's both a literal and metaphorical threshold they are crossing. The tracks represent a physical path away from their home. And once they embark on their adventure, the boys are crossing the threshold from boyhood to adulthood.

These moments within stories allow the reader or audience to switch their own mindsets, knowing that the characters are going to be facing the central conflict, as well as many challenges throughout their journey. The is usually the most engaging moment in the story.

DOI: 10.4324/9781003182009-6

The threshold of the Special or Other World is the world that the hero is about to encounter as he meets the Call he's been forced to – or has chosen to – accept. And it's essential that the story presents a world that is very different, fantasy-like, from the one the hero is used to. In *Stand By Me*, when the boys embark on their adventure, there are no parents to guide them, and they've escaped the constraints of their life in Castle Rock. It's just them, the tracks, a long and intimidating bridge, a murky swamp and the coming-of-age conflicts and realisations that comprise the new world they've entered.

In *The Lord of the Rings*, the hobbits are in a dark, strange and dangerous world. Everyone is bigger than they are. They don't know who to trust. And they certainly don't have enough food. They're out of their comfort zone.

The threshold represents the difference between the known and the unknown. In Sunderland's book *A Pea Called Mildred* (1999), Mildred is a pea with dreams. She has great plans for her pea life. However, people are always telling her that dreams are pointless as she is just another ordinary pea. Eventually, with the help of a kind person along the way, Mildred ends up doing exactly what she has always dreamed of doing and opens a tea shop. In the real world, we perceive a pea as just a pea. Yet in the fantasy of the Other World, the pea becomes a symbol that can inspire children to dream. Using metaphor allows the children to enter into the realm of their imagination where anything becomes possible. Mildred crosses the threshold when she realises that her fantasy is possible.

When children approach the crossing the threshold stage, you can facilitate this for them by introducing a dramatic context. This allows them to act out this stage through character, metaphor and story. A good group exercise here is building a rocket ship, which I have outlined for you in Chapter 8.

Other times, they will shift naturally through this stage, but this is rare.

Case study

AM – do you see me as I see myself?

AM was 9 years of age, the youngest of three sisters. She was struggling to find her voice in her family. Through her play we identified that she felt different from her siblings and misunderstood by her family generally. She was quick to anger, and her family struggled to like her. AM was blamed for being the one to spoil the family fun with her 'drama'. She was seen as the problem. AM was a hard client for me to like, too. She didn't give much away during her sessions, and building a relationship took time. What changed everything was when her parents came into her session towards the end of her therapy. She had requested that both of them attend. AM's favourite game was making potions, specifically slime. This is messy, so I set the ingredients out on the table where AM usually sat to make her slime. As her parents got stuck into making the slime with her, following her instructions, she visibly changed before my eyes. She smiled at both of her parents and directed them in a relaxed way. Her father literally rolled up his sleeves and mixed the dry and wet ingredients together. Her mother told me afterwards that they hadn't seen AM behave with them like this before. There was no anger. In that game she introduced them to a side of her they hadn't seen before. Instead of showing them her anger, she expressed her joyful feelings about making and holding the slime – something they found disgusting – creating something from start to finish. An important stage in AM's slime-making was the final act where she poured the slime into a small container with a lid. Securing the lid onto the container and enclosing the slime represented AM being able to contain and hold her own feelings, something she had been struggling to find a comfortable way to do. During the session, her mother admitted that she wasn't allowed to make slime at home because it was too messy and AM got it 'everywhere'. For the first time in her life, her parents were witnessing AM's joyful messy world, and taking part in it, without judgement. AM had crossed the threshold and shown them exactly what she needed from them, the chance to be creative without judgement, in a way that made sense to her, and for them to witness her mess. When children receive this unconditional support and acknowledgement it makes them feel accepted and loved. This is what helps to build their confidence and self-esteem.

Theoretical background – understanding creation being a messenger of meaning

The exercise I have chosen for this lesson expands on the concept of moulding/self-reflection, and invites children to form the shape of themselves in the clay.

Clay therapy explains how clients can touch that sacred part of themselves that might have been shut down through trauma.

By using clay therapeutically I will know more about myself and my clients because working with clay helps us to access hidden thoughts and touch our unconscious material. Clay does not lie. James Hillman (1997) refers to the idea of the creation being a messenger of meaning, and how we can learn from that if we take the time to ponder on the clay form.

By listening to my intuition and witnessing, I can be in tune with the client and therefore work with a deeper level of empathy and understanding so that I can make a 'knowing contact' with them.

By seeing the therapy session like an archaeologist's dig, I will be able to help clients move from the surface to deeper personal levels as our psyches make connections with the clay creations, and a narrative emerges which is a personal story. (This approach is similar to the way I work therapeutically with adults through art and words to find a personal story and voice that unites body, mind and soul into one narrative.)

When playing with metaphors, more brain centres light up in response to metaphor than any other form of human communication, forming new neural pathways.

If I surrender to the process the unknown will emerge.

A psychological touching provides a deeper psychological contact than opioids and oxytocin hormones that gives us a sense of wellbeing are released in the brain, providing an inner feeling of calmness and peacefulness. Sunderland (2003) calls this 'hormonal heaven'.

Working therapeutically with clay is a journey taken at the client's pace, although there are times when it is appropriate to be more directive, for example when exploring anger issues.

Combining the use of musical instruments followed by clay can enable the client to connect with their unexpressed anger.

When dealing with medical and health concerns, the story that emerges through the clay belongs to the clay, which makes it emotionally safer to speak about.

Souter-Anderson (2010) describes clay as being fundamental, like the earth. Touching the clay is touching the sacred, like touching the soul because the pot that is formed is like the body, it's a container for the soul. Therefore working with clay is like working with what Jung calls the 'captive world-soul'.

Souter-Anderson is the client's 'emotional midwife', holding the client's suffering while they transform it through the process of working in relationship with the therapist and with clay.

The research is taken directly from Souter-Anderson's book, *Touching Clay, Touching What? The Use of Clay in Therapy* (2010), which focused on locating the bridging concepts that illuminate what makes working therapeutically with clay valuable.

This research led Souter-Anderson to create a theoretical underpinning of clay in therapy which draws on Jungian theory and Object Relations theories. These place the focus on what goes on between the client, the therapist and the clay and the emerging existential theme which is an expression of the client's unconscious experience, and the final outcome of therapeutic clay work.

Souter-Anderson's (2010) 'Theory of Contact' is anchored in five lenses for therapeutic clay work. All five lenses work simultaneously in the therapy and come into focus like a kaleidoscope:

1. Making contact with the clay and the primal self begins the birthing stage of a process.
2. Play Space of Potential – through touching the clay, body and mind work in an integrated way which can move the client to experience an altered state of consciousness.
3. Clay play in the presence of another – the emotional contact with the clay and the therapist encourages the client to explore. In this transitional space the clay becomes a transitional object which acts as a bridge between the outer and inner worlds of the client.
4. Bridging space of potential – the relationship between therapist and client is 'the vessel where vaporisation of an understanding can be distilled'. As an 'emotional midwife', the therapist waits to 'catch and hold the narration' (Souter-Anderson, 2010) so that the client feels safe to play and engage with their imagination, and let the metaphorical and symbolic images emerge.

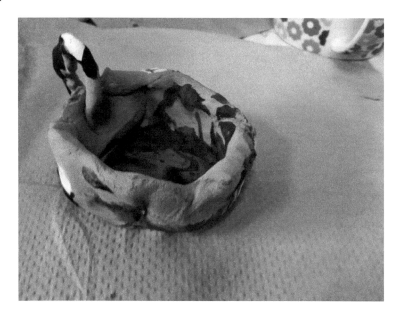

Figure 4.1 Clay container.

5. Emerging theme – an existential theme emerges through an exploration of the image. Examples of existential themes are covered in case studies from Souter-Anderson's research. The themes are grouped into four world views, described by Heidegger, Binswanger (1946) and May (1994) as: *Umwelt* (Earth), *Mitwelt* (World), *Eigenwelt* (Man) and *Uberwelt* (Gods) and the Four Dimensions of Human Experience Model, reframed by van Deurzen as: the physical dimension (Life/Death), social dimension (Love/Hate), personal dimension (Strength/Weakness) and spiritual dimension (Good/Evil).

Souter-Anderson shows us how exploration is a creative and illuminating process that unfolds in a 'kaleidoscopic pattern' if the therapist and client play together.

Lesson plan: make a clay object of a gargoyle, alien or monster

Overview
    In this lesson, students explore their identity in relation to the concept of the earth through clay.
Recommended age group
    Education providers for ages KS1 and KS2.
Time
    55 minutes approximately.
Equipment
    Clay.
    Wire cutter.

Oilcloth/heavy duty plastic/vinyl mat to protect the floor or space.

Small wooden boards to place the lump of clay on and mould.

Various sizes of polythene container.

Plastic bottle for holding water to wet the clay.

Bucket for putting clay creations no longer wanted in.

Dustpan and brush.

Hand wipes.

Some tools for modelling – small rolling pins, blunt plastic knives, small stones and shells, pegs.

Preparation

Hand out a wooden board and lump of clay to each child.

Give them 15 minutes to create a gargoyle, alien or monster.

The moulding of these forms is helpful in exploring:

- Fears, worries and anxieties.
- Ways of fending off fears, worries and anxieties.
- Anger.

Confidence to work with clay

If you are nervous about how best to start working with clay, my advice is to play with the clay yourself first before introducing this into your class. Give yourself permission to connect with your inner child, recall a time when your enjoyed playing, and go for it! If you are concerned about the messiness of the clay, be curious about what that might be about.

Questions to ask the class

Ask the class to write their answers to the following questions on their paper plates:

Titling: invite the children to think of a title for their clay object.

Story: invite the children to tell you the story of their clay form. Or they can write this on the back of their paper plate.

Ask the children if they want to take the object home. If they don't, give them the choice to dispose of the object in the bucket.

Interpretation

We don't want to move too deeply into interpreting these objects. What we do want to listen out for is the possible use of metaphor. This will give us clues as to what the child is trying to communicate through the clay object. Some of this may be revealing and noteworthy.

Observe if there are any changes in the children's physical movements, facial expressions or breathing. It is likely they are connecting to some emotion.

Classroom tips

Identify students for whom this topic may be challenging

Children and young people with disabilities or who have experienced abuse, extreme trauma, bereavement or themselves suffer with a mental health condition may find discussions about home and relationships quite challenging. It is important to be aware of these students before teaching this lesson and of any sensitivities or issues that may come up.

Teacher skill – active containing and reflecting the children's feelings back to them

When I hear parents say to me 'My child is running rings around me', this tells me that the child does not feel contained in the relationship. A boundary is being broken to enable the child to do this. Perhaps the child feels those boundaries are too restrictive for their self-expression and is showing their disapproval to try and get more room, space to be expressive. Whatever the reason, containment is an important factor in a child's sense of feeling safe in the relationship. Containment is interesting because the quality of it will depend on how contained the adult feels, so it's always worth doing a routine check-in with yourself if you find yourself in that situation. If you find yourself feeling triggered by the child's behaviour, it is likely that part of you is not feeling contained.

If we are comfortable containing the energy of a child's play in all its manifestations we will communicate this to them, without words, in our manner, our way of inviting them to play and our intentions. Our containing needs to be modulated even in our own body sense by each particular child and their needs. Our active containing often serves as a ground wire for the child's emotional and energetic surges and as the ground itself for the leaping is play. The space itself is a part of the containment, and most of the materials serve as part of the containment as well. I find that children are quite relieved when they feel adequately contained (McCarthy, 2012, p. 33).

Here is a short containment exercise you can do if you start to feel wobbly and triggered, which will help to calm your nervous system so that you start to feel more regulated.

Close your eyes and visualize your safe place. In this safe place you are going to place your container. This can either be a small box, a safe or a vault. Open this container and place your worries inside it. Name each worry as you place it inside your container. Close the lid of the container and lock it. Put the key in your pocket. Leave the container in your safe place and open your eyes.

References

Binswinger, L. (1946). 'The existential analysis school of thought'. In R. May et al. (eds) *Existence*. New York: Basic Books.

Hillman, J. (1997). *Suicide and the Soul*. Woodstock, CT: Spring Publications.

McCarthy, D. (2012). *A Manual of Dynamic Play Therapy: Helping Things Fall Apart, the Paradox of Play*. London: Jessica Kingsley Publishers.

Souter-Anderson, L. (2010). *Touching Clay, Touching What? The Use of Clay in Therapy*. Dorset: Archive Publishing.

Sunderland, M. (1999). *A Pea Called Mildred: A Story to Help Children Pursue Their Hopes and Dreams*. Oxford: Speechmark Publishing.

Sunderland, M. (2003). *Using Story Telling as a Therapeutic Tool with Children*. Oxford: Speechmark Publishing.

Chapter 5

Finding allies and enemies

Introduction

The hero learns the rules of his new world. During this time, he endure tests of strength of will, meets friends and comes face to face with enemies. The period in his journey helps him define his relationship with other characters in the story. During this part of the journey, he learns who will help him and who will hinder him.

This is the stage where children face their fears, and discover how they can overcome them. They do this through discovering characters in the story who represent those allies (strengths) and enemies (fears).

This delicate stage in the process is supported by the adult who learns how to listen attentively to the child's process, handle the questions raised by the child and reflect back to the child what they are hearing. This all helps the child to see and understand the capacity they have to solve their own problems, without external interventions.

You will recognise children who are at this stage in their journey. They may be experiencing relationship difficulties with their peers, bullying or isolation may be a problem for them.

Case study

OH and PH – will you be my lockdown buddy?

This case study was undertaken during lockdown. It was completed at a physical distance via Zoom. Surprisingly, the context of distance and

DOI: 10.4324/9781003182009-7

technology created both a narrowing and a laser-like quality to the interview. For compatibility with these qualities I chose the 6PSM (6-Part Story-making Method) which I have adapted as the creative medium. Initially I was concerned about the brevity of this case study but, on reflection, I see how each of the six boxes packs a punch, and is an opportunity to go deeper into the story, at some point. The story told here is complete in itself, and reflects just how much ground was actually covered during lockdown, how children were running heroic emotional marathons every day.

The 6 box story templates were emailed to the parents in advance of the Zoom meeting. I had explained the nature and format of the questions I would be asking to the parents. I would invite the children to draw a picture in each box in response to my questions. I would write any notes into a 6 box story template to complement the drawings. These allowed me to reflect on the drawings after the session. Their Mum sat alongside both OL and TL during their interviews.

Every child will have their own lockdown story which reflects their circumstances and experience. The 6 box story is a good starting point for telling these stories, and for using them as an assessment tool for coping mechanisms and resilience.

Once upon a time, there was a character called xxx.
Draw a picture of your character.

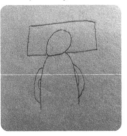

Their mission was to 'stay at home' and not catch a virus.
Draw a picture of this mission.

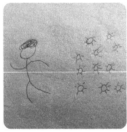

The most difficult part about this mission was xxx.
Draw this difficulty.

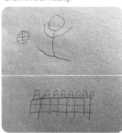

Some people helped xxx to cope.
Draw what that help felt like.

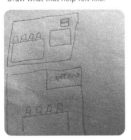

Xxx learned stuff about himself and the mission.
Draw what you learned.

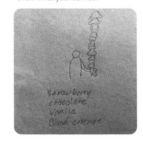

If you had another mission what would you take with you?.
Draw this.

Figure 5.1 Ice Cream Bot 3000: OH's 6 box story.

OH is 8 years old. He lives with his Mum, Dad and younger sister PH. They went through lockdown together in the same house, their home. OH reached this stage during lockdown. He completed the story template in six boxes. The lockdown showed OH a different side of his sister who he described as usually being 'grouchy'. During lockdown he said she 'got funnier' and became an ally. He missed seeing his friends, and learnt to use his Nintendo Switch to change focus when he got stressed. He said that if he had to undertake another mission like lockdown, he would take his friends and family with him, along with his ice-cream maker, Nintendo Switch, Covid testing kit (just in case) and an Rubik's cube to challenge his mind. He would carry all this in his backpack. When I asked him how this felt, he described it as feeling 'heavy and rough', but he said that he wouldn't be carrying this heavy load all by himself, his family and friends would take turns to carry it.

It seemed to me that OH had access to resources: family and activities to keep him busy and occupied; he used his imagination to read *Harry Potter* whereas pre-pandemic he had been more interested in playing football. Although he saw the pandemic as an enemy because it stopped him from seeing his friends and going to school, he discovered that his sister became his close ally. Thrown together for company, his Mum told me that during the lockdown she noticed OH and his sister lying on the floor of

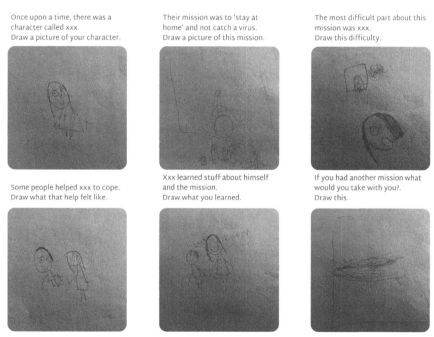

Once upon a time, there was a character called xxx.
Draw a picture of your character.

Their mission was to 'stay at home' and not catch a virus.
Draw a picture of this mission.

The most difficult part about this mission was xxx.
Draw this difficulty.

Some people helped xxx to cope.
Draw what that help felt like.

Xxx learned stuff about himself and the mission.
Draw what you learned.

If you had another mission what would you take with you?.
Draw this.

Figure 5.2 Unicorn Magic Cake: PH's 6 box story.

their bedroom, talking quietly. This was something they hadn't been doing pre-pandemic. They were more likely to play alone or with their friends. She overheard them whispering to each other, and found this new-found intimacy and connection between them to be a positive sign of their developing relationship.

PH's story, shown in Figure 5.2, reflects a similar narrative. She discovered her brother, Mum and Dad helped her to get unstuck by explaining things to her. She also learned to ask for help, and if she had to undertake another mission, she wanted to take some cake with her!

Theoretical background – understanding the dramatic and therapeutic potential of story making

I became aware of the work of Professor Mooli Lahad, an educational psychologist and director of the MA studies in Dramatherapy at Tel Hai College, Israel in 2011. He created the BASIC 'Ph Model' of Coping and Resilience in the wake of both natural and man-made disasters. He worked closely with Alida Gersie on her 6-Part Story-making Method (6PSM). This is a creative format of making up stories and exploring their dramatic and therapeutic potential for individuals and groups (Shacham and Lahad, 2012, p. 47). Lahad and Gersie noticed during their 5-year collaboration that the invented stories revealed the students' ways of coping which corresponded with Lahad's model of resiliency. After completing training in 6PSM, I decided to introduce the 6PSM to outpatients at Great Ormond Street Hospital (GOSH). The results were astonishing and can be applied in the school environment, too. I did, however, make some adaptations of my own to 6PSM, to tailor it for the hospital environment. I particularly liked 6PSM because stories told in 6PSM are based on a hero-quest sequence which is easy to explain to children, given the vast number of comic-book heroes now available on film! The moment you mention the word 'hero' or 'superhero' to children, they get the significance of what you are asking them to imagine, and quickly dive into their collection of stories. Jung et al. (1964), researchers of fairy tales and stories based on a Jungian approach, found that the answers to six questions can always be found in fairy tales. These six questions are used as the story structure in 6PSM:

- Who is (are) the main character/s (hero/heroine)?
- What is the task or mission of the main character/s?
- Who or what can help (if at all)?
- What is the obstacle in the way or what prevents the task from happening?
- How does/do the main character/s cope with the problem?
- What happens next or how does the story end?

Listening to the child's needs

You might be wondering what the criteria are for using or creating a therapeutic story, and a framework like 6PSM. The key is to listen to the child's needs, and to create the story around them. Identify a theme. Erickson views symptom as a message or 'gift' (Mills and Crowley, 1986, p. 45) from the unconscious that can be used to resolve the symptom. At the heart of Erickson's approach is a philosophy of acceptance and validation of the child's presenting behaviour (Mills and Crowley, 1986, p. 47) which is consistent with Axline's second principle of accepting the child exactly as they are. Erickson's technique of utilisation also requires professionals to be skilled in observing, participating in and reframing what the child presents in the clinical situation (Mills and Crowley, 1986, p. 48). For example, if the child has a great deal of energy, match that energy by choosing very energetic kangaroos or monkeys as story characters because they will identify with their energy level.

Mellon refers to the 'Four Elements' guidelines that have helped her to create and organise stories. 'If your child is full of fire, and stomps about the house, then you need not waste your time with a story about a little gerbil …' (Mellon, 2000, p. 57). Similarly, children who are more connected to air than fire, who leap lightly about on their toes, respond to lilting stories filled with bright birds.

Next we can start to develop a strategy and story framework and put the chosen issues into a metaphorical context to which we know the child will relate. The key here is to choose an idea from a story source we know, a literary metaphor, a fictional metaphor, a fairy tale, a myth or a story drawn from our own experience. This is where the character we choose as our protagonist will share the same emotional problem – metaphorical conflict – as the child. This is when we need to know the emotional themes that recur in the child's play (Sunderland, 2003, p. 23) so that the journey the child will go on through the story will be the same as their own, and they will be able to identify with the character's defeats and obstacles, and ultimately feel the character's triumph.

This is how empathy gets through to the child (Sunderland, 2003, p. 16). For example, one of my clients had an issue with being the only mixed-race child in the school, and had feelings of not belonging. I chose a fantastical context – a teapot called Tilly who was born in a pot factory, and who is the only teapot with a crinkly spout. This provided the protection of disguise and indirect expression for my client which allowed her to explore her feelings through this metaphorical fantasy. It is through fantasy that the child learns to make sense of their outside world (Mills and Crowley, 1986, p. 36). This metaphor helped me to change the literal into the symbolic for my client. As Sunderland says, sometimes the more 'dotty' the better (Sunderland, 2003, p. 25). By creating this metaphor I had also created a three-way empathic relationship between the child, therapist and story, which made it possible for the child to develop a sense of identification with the characters and events of the metaphor. It is this sense of identification that contains the transformational power of the metaphor (Gordon (1978) in Mills and Crowley, 1986, p. 65) as I witnessed after I read this story to my client.

As Combs and Freedman state (1990, p. 45), our clients tell us where to look to create metaphors. We learn this by entering our client's world of thinking, feeling and the unconscious, and by listening and paying attention to what they tell us and how they move, behave and play. And, finally, we use symbols to gather information about our client's mood and intentions. Professionals in the classroom are in a unique position to be aware of these stories and to discover story metaphors within them.

Lesson plan: the 6 box story

Overview
> In this lesson, students explore the concept of finding allies and enemies by completing the 6 box story.

Recommended age group
> Education providers for ages KS1 and KS2.

Time
> 55 minutes approximately.

Equipment
> Blank 6 box story templates.
> Coloured crayons.

Preparation
> What you will need:
> The 6 box story templates.
> Then in each box write the appropriate question. I ask the question and invite the children to draw their answer in each box. As the story continues and develops the children usually get completely absorbed in telling it and their energy and movement changes. This is how you know they are making connections with their own story. When the story is finished, this is your opportunity to reflect on how the children are/are not coping which will help you decide on the intervention possibilities.
> Teachers can use this exercise with children as an assessment tool to use prior to making a therapeutic referral. You may find that completing this exercise is enough for the child.

Questions to ask yourself during reflection
- Does this story suggest an intervention that is balancing, helping the child to 'bounce back'?
- Is the story about regaining strengths and separating from the teacher after a short and focused encounter?
- Does the story show very few coping resources or too many channels in conflict? If so, then a longer therapy may be indicated.
- Does the story reveal developmental concerns and conflicts that belong to a very young age or are not at all age appropriate?
- Are the character's problems chronic or is the quest circular, so that a supportive approach may be the most suitable recommendation?

Questions to ask the class
> When they have completed the exercise, ask the class to tell you about it, and use their answers as prompts to explore what resources they are missing. Listen attentively to what troubles/disturbs/upsets them, and explore this sensitively with them. Take this as far as they want to take it. Always take your cue from them.

Interpretation

We don't want to move too deeply into interpreting these objects. What we do want to listen out for are the possible uses of metaphor. This will give us clues as to what the child is trying to communicate through the story. Some of this may be revealing and noteworthy. Be aware if there are any changes in the children's physical movements, facial expressions or breathing. It is likely they are connecting to some emotion.

Classroom tips

Identify students for whom this topic may be challenging

Children and young people with disabilities or who have experienced abuse, extreme trauma, bereavement or themselves suffer with a mental health condition may find discussions around home and relationships quite challenging. It is important to be aware of these students before teaching this lesson and of any sensitivities or issues that may come up.

Teacher skill: active listening to attune to the child's solutions to their problems

Resistance can often be fear disguised. Fear of revealing a secret. Fear of being vulnerable. Fear of getting into trouble. You don't want to unpack this too much, in order to avoid doing so when you encounter resistance, move swiftly and invite the child to draw the feeling. This will help them to contain their feelings. You can then use the drawing as a talking point to move further through the resistance.

What we need to do is to acknowledge the child is struggling and accept the pain this is causing them, and we do this by doing what Carl Rogers called 'active listening' (Kirschenbaum and Henderson, 1990). So in the midst of a struggle, we can start by asking children questions, such as: 'What do you need from me right now, in this situation?' And then wait for the answer! 'Active listening' is an important way to bring about changes in people. Despite the popular notion that listening is a passive approach, clinical and research evidence clearly shows that sensitive listening is a most effective agent for individual personality change and group development.

Active listening requires the listener to concentrate fully, understand, respond and then remember what has being said. This is opposed to reflective listening where the listener repeats back to the speaker what they have just heard to confirm understanding of both parties.

I use active listening in my work with families, especially parents who are at the end of their patience with their child's ramped-up behaviour. I usually start by asking them: 'What do you think your child is trying to tell you based on what you hear?' Nine times out of ten the parents are shocked when we have drilled down on this question to find what the child is really trying to say! Once they have 'got it', parents are more equipped to cope with the ups and downs of their child's emotions. Active listening is particularly challenging for busy, stressed parents and teachers because so often they are operating in 'fix-it' mode which is all about taking action. We need to find a way to slow things down during communication so that we can actively listen and hear what the children are saying or communicating through their behaviour.

Patty Wipfler and Tosha Schore, authors of the book *Listen: Five Simple Tools to Meet Your Everyday Parenting Challenges* (2016), call this practice 'stay listen-ing' which means listening all the way through your child's upset. If your child is crying, stay with them instead of giving them a fix-it solution: 'If you stop crying we can go and get ice-cream', for example.

I know that it can be tough to slow down communication in a busy classroom which is why I hope using the 6 box story template will be a useful tool for when there is time outside the classroom to spend one-to-one with the child. In most cases, the most useful tool will be the three As:

- Acknowledge the child's feelings first.
- Accept the child exactly as they are.
- Agree any action last, with the child's consent.

References

Combs, G. and Freedman, J. (1990). *Symbol, Story and Ceremony: Using Metaphor in Individual and Family Therapy*. New York: W.W. Norton & Company, Inc.

Jung, C.J., von Franz, M.-L., Henderson, Joseph L., Jaffe, A. and Jacobi, J. (1964). *Man and His Symbols*. New York: Doubleday.

Kirschenbaum, H. and Henderson, V.L. (eds) (1990). *The Carl Rogers Reader. Reflections from the Lifetime Work of America's Preeminent Psychologist*. London: Constable.

Mellon, N. (2000). *Storytelling with Children*. Stroud: Hawthorn Press.

Mills, J.C. and Crowley, R. (1986). *Therapeutic Metaphors for Children and the Child Within*. London: Brunner-Routledge.

Shacham, M. and Lahad. O.A.M. (2012). *The 'BASIC Ph' Model of Coping and Resilience: Theory, Research and Cross-Cultural Application*. London: Jessica Kingsley Publishers.

Sunderland, M. (2003). *Using Story Telling as a Therapeutic Tool with Children*. Oxford: Speechmark Publishing.

Wipfler, P. and Schore, T. (2016). *Listen: Five Simple Tools to Meet Your Everyday Parenting Challenges*. Palo Alto, CA: Hand in Hand Parenting.

Chapter 6

Revelation

Introduction

The hero has survived death, overcome his greatest fear, slain the dragon or weathered the Crisis of the Heart, and his reward comes in different forms: a magical sword, an elixir, greater knowledge or insight, reconciliation with a friend or family member. The hero has learned what he needs to overcome his challenge, and feels more hopeful and optimistic about his own agency to cope with the changes he faces.

This proves to the child, and the adult, what their resilience looks and feels like.

Case study

ERS – I know the answer!

This is a review of three sandtrays made by a 6-year-old boy called ERS, referred to me for 24 play therapy sessions following his adoption. His presenting issue was his angry outbursts, whereas his underlying issue concerned his ambivalence about being adopted. The client was adopted out of foster care together with his younger sister by a childless couple. Both children had been badly neglected and emotionally and physically abused by their birth parents. The children had lived with a foster family for two years, which had been a settled placement. These sandtrays were created during the first 12 of 24 sessions at Catmose Primary School, Oakham. The sandtray conformed to European tray size standard 49.5 x 72 x 7.5 cm, and was painted blue on the bottom to represent water. I sat alongside ERS while he created his sandtrays. ERS left his sessions with the sandplay

---

intact, which enabled him to carry the images with him. Once he had left his sessions, I photographed the sandtrays, before dismantling them. The sandplay was non-directed in that the client decided on the expression of his therapeutic sand process.

Theoretical background – understanding sandplay as a therapeutic method that facilitates the psyche's natural capacity for healing

Sandplay is hands-on psychological work, and is an adjunct to talk therapy. It is a powerful therapeutic method that facilitates the psyche's natural capacity for healing.

John Daly (1987) says that the psyche contains a fundamental, autonomous tendency (drive) towards self-healing and wholeness, and has the tendency to balance itself through the compensatory functions of the unconscious. The process of creative imagination in sandplay provides a method of connecting the world of ego consciousness with the deepest realms of the psyche – the archetypal and transpersonal worlds. This results in a more natural balance developing between the ego-orientated intellect and the true Self. There is a re-aligning and balancing of the masculine and feminine aspects of the psyche giving the client a more holistic and balanced world view. In the sandplay, we see the client's story created as a concrete manifestation from their imagination using sand and miniature objects. Sandplay helps illuminate the client's internal symbolic world, providing a place for its expression within the safe container of the sandtray and the therapeutic relationship.

Sandplay 1

I felt very drawn to this sandplay because of the point of conflict between the red emergency vehicle and the magic wand. They appear to symbolise two opposing energetic principles of being rescued and empowered, and I wondered if they symbolised ERS's ambivalent feelings about his removal from his foster care parents, and subsequent placement with adoptive parents. ERS expressed his anger by ramming the emergency vehicle into the sandtray, and then abandoned it when the wheels failed to turn round in the sand. Before putting the vehicle in the upright position, he had crashed it on its side and covered it with sand, which explains the sand still on the left-hand side of the vehicle. While he was enacting this scene he was making loud grunting noises.

Placing of objects

Different theorists have different theories about the significance of symbols, and where they may be placed in the sandtray. In sandplay 1, there is no central core of objects in the sandtray. The objects give the appearance of being randomly placed, with the emergency vehicle placed on the diagonal left and the wand placed on the diagonal right. I wonder if their placement reflects the two opposing sides of the client's left rational brain and his right creative brain. The fallen Knight lies on his back at the side of the vehicle, and standing on top of the vehicle is the superhero Hulk character.

Symbolism of the objects

> The meaning of these images cannot be fully understood by the intellect, but it can be experienced and known by the psyche as a whole.
>
> (Jung, 1958)

The objects and images are symbols that function as a means of releasing sources of energy from the unconscious (Chetwynd, 1982). Decoding the symbols gives us clues to possible intended meanings. Only the child knows what these objects and images mean because what functions as a symbol for one child may function as a sign for another. The symbol offers an opportunity for a new way of addressing a crisis (Turner, 2005, p. 38).

Daly (1987) says that for boys in Neumann's warlike stages crashed trucks can symbolise powerful aggressive tendencies. The truck's control panel is outside the sandtray because ERS threw it down on the floor when the wheels stopped turning in the sand. I wonder about the meaning of this metaphor. The control panel cable can be seen in the sandtray, which makes me feel that ERS's sense of control is outside himself, and perhaps that is one reason why he needs to express his aggressive feelings towards his adopted mother.

Tressider (2003, p. 372) says the magic wand is linked to fairy tales which influence the future by making wishes come true. The Fairy Godmother's Wand is a powerful magical tool, capable of various enchanting abilities, such as conjuration, metamorphosis (turning Cinderella's rags into a ballgown, the glass coach into a pumpkin), enchantment and time manipulation. Bettelheim (1975, p. 52) says as long as a child remains unsure that their immediate human environment will protect them, they need to believe that superior powers, such as a guardian angel, watch over them. It is therefore possible that the placing of the wand in the sandtray symbolises ERS's wishful thinking, and perhaps hope, that the difficult aspects in his life will magically improve, or at least counter the Hulk's superhero powers.

There is a fallen Knight lying next to the emergency truck, which symbolizes the fallen hero, and I wonder if this represents ERS's biological father who eventually abandoned him and his sister. ERS developed a close relationship with his foster father, and I wonder whether aspects of him falling from grace by giving ERS up for adoption are also symbolised in this object. The superhero Hulk object symbolises superhuman power and strength, and an ability to crush any opposing force. Here he represents the glory of having won the battle against the Knight, but his characteristic use of brute force suggests a *negative dynamic masculine* archetype (Hill, 1992, p.12). The negative aspects of the dynamic masculine are its excess and drive to dominate and its failure to recognise or acknowledge any other point of view, so that the creative thrust is 'perverted into destructiveness' (Hill, 1992, p.12) expressed through directed violence, a disregard for nature and the ecological

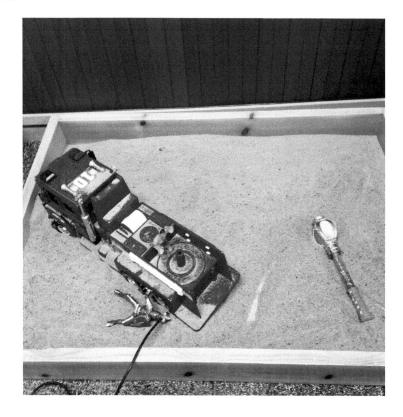

Figure 6.1 **Sandplay 1.**

consequences of one's actions. ERS's early life experience with his biological parents was unsafe and unboundaried, with violent outbursts from his biological father. ERS's male role models abused him and abandoned him, leaving ERS with a lot of rage and a need for both superhero strength and a magic wand's powers to neutralise the *negative dynamic masculine* archetype. There is no evidence in this sandplay of the *static feminine* archetype, the great nurturing Mother.

In between the truck and the wand, we can see some blue of the bottom of the sandtray, which symbolises the unconscious. ERS talked very little while making his sandplay, which is consistent with this small revelation of blue.

The sand in the sandtray looks relatively undisturbed, indicative perhaps of the fact that ERS feels secure enough to express his aggression. There is nothing central, animated or populated about this tray, nothing pulling me into the world of ERS. The energy focus in this tray is of polar opposites and the overall feeling is of stark contrasts and choices.

Sandplay 2

This sandplay was created the week following sandplay 1. The energy focus in this sandplay is with the Action Man object, lying inert in the top right-hand corner

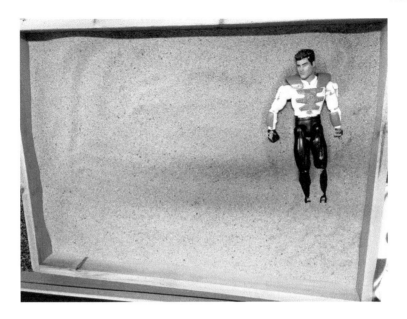

Figure 6.2 **Sandplay 2.**

of the sandtray. ERS buried him first, and then uncovered him. Although there is no core to this tray or point of conflict, this symbol does seem to embody ERS's need to be powerful, and this symbol reflects the masculine archetype of the hero. Hill (1992, p.10) describes four patterns of individual intrapsychic modes of consciousness and the *dynamic masculine* is expressed in the archetypal image of the Dragon-Slaying Hero and the drive to conquer and slay the 'devouring aspects of the *static feminine*'. The dynamic masculine is only interested in achieving its goal and is characterised by serving its own ambition and initiative. This reflects ERS's behaviour at home where he was driven to win board games at all costs and lost his temper if he didn't win, becoming aggressive and sometimes violent towards his mother. The absence of any female archetypal symbol suggests that the masculine is being developed at the expense of the feminine (Bradway and McCoard, 2010, p. 188).

Sandplay 3

This sandplay is made up exclusively of animal life which is typical of Kalf's animal-vegetative stage of ego development (Bradway and McCoard, 2010, p. 110). The lizard is pre-historic and forms the core centre of this sandplay. ERS used the lizard symbol for six weeks in the sandplay, and created other lizard objects in other media (painting, drawing, clay and paper). He drew lizards first, and then cut them out to keep in his special box. We made the clay Godzilla together, which he painted green. Several of these objects were kept in his special box.

The lizard represented ERS's primal rage and mistrust of human life; he enacted scenes of attack and defended himself using the lizard.

The energy focus of this tray feels predatory, the lizard looks poised to attack even though it's the only object in the sandplay. ERS used the magic wand to drag through the sand and form the circle around the lizard, creating a boundary to contain the lizard and perhaps his own primal feelings, which sometimes overwhelmed him during the sessions.

Lesson plan: making a sandtray of your inner wisdom

Overview
   In this lesson, students explore the concept of discovering their inner wisdom through sandplay objects.
Recommended age group
   Education providers for ages KS1 and KS2.
Time
   55 minutes approximately.
Equipment
   Sandtray (or washing up bowl).
   Sand.
   Selection of objects including mystical characters, urns, trees, wand, swords.
Preparation
   Pour the sand into the tray or bowl and smooth it out so that the surface is as flat as you can get it.
   Place the objects on a table alongside the tray or bowl.
   Invite the children to choose three objects and place them in the sand.
   Give the children a few minutes to arrange the objects and get comfortable with the process. It won't be long before they start to tell you about their objects. Encourage them to tell you the story. Remember this isn't about you critiquing them, it's about you witnessing them. Be alert for clues.
Questions to ask yourself during reflection
   - Does this story suggest an intervention that is balancing, helping the child to 'bounce back'?
   - Is it about regaining strengths and separating from the teacher after a short and focused encounter?
   - Does the story show very few coping resources or too many channels in conflict? If so, then a longer therapy may be indicated.
   - Does the story reveal developmental concerns and conflicts that belong to a very young age or are not at all age appropriate?
   - Are the character's problems chronic, or is the quest circular, so that a supportive approach may be the most suitable recommendation?
Questions to ask the class
   When the children have completed the exercise, ask them to tell you about it and use their answers as prompts to explore what resources they are missing. Listen attentively to what troubles/disturbs/upsets them, and explore this sensitively with them. Take this as far as they want to take it. Always take your cue from them.

Interpretation

We don't want to move too deeply into interpreting these objects. What we do want to listen out for are the possible uses of metaphor. This will give us clues as to what the child is trying to communicate through the clay object. Some of this may be revealing and noteworthy. Be aware if there are any changes in the children's physical movements, facial expressions or breathing. It is likely they are connecting to some emotion.

Classroom tips

Identify students for whom this topic may be challenging

Children and young people with disabilities or who have experienced abuse, extreme trauma, bereavement or themselves suffer with a mental health condition may find discussions around home and relationships quite challenging. It is important to be aware of these students before teaching this lesson and of any sensitivities or issues that may come up.

Teacher skill – becoming non-directive: the teacher does not attempt to direct the child's play or conversation, the child leads the way, the teacher follows

When I first learnt this skill during my play therapy training, I had to sit on my hands to remind myself not to offer praise or suggestions! Both of these must be excluded from your repertoire. If you fall into the trap of offering praise, the child will see this as an inducement to act in a certain manner in order to receive more praise. If the child asks for your help, you must give it, and if they ask you for any specific help with using the materials, you must give that as well. If the child is making a sandtray, you do not suggest that they move or reposition a certain object in a different place. It must be their choice where they place their objects.

In this context, you must be clear about your role. You are not the teacher, playmate or substitute mother. You are a sounding board against which the child can test their personality. You are the one who holds up the mirror so that they can see themself exactly as they are. You must keep your personal opinions, feelings and guidance to yourself. This is where the self-help toolkit will help you.

This is how the child starts to trust themself. The more you take yourself out of the equation, the more freedom they will have to bring themself into it. This can be quite challenging at first for some children, so be prepared for them to ask you for directions. When they do this, make sure to keep your guidance focused on the materials. Use your reflection skills as in this example:

Child: You see my father and mother aren't any relation any more. They are divorced and father is married again. (He sighs deeply and closes the paint box with a bang. He goes over to the shelf and picks up the nursing bottle. He sucks on it.)
Child: Me baby.

Therapist: You could be their baby.
>   (Child picks up the draughts game and brings it back to the table and sits down across from the therapist.)

Child: You play with me.
>   (The draughts are placed on the board and a conventional game of draughts begins. Halfway through the game the child tells the therapist what draught to move and where to put it.)

Therapist: You want to tell me what to do in this game.

Child: Yes. Look. This is how I want you to play.

Therapist: You want to tell me what to do.

Child: Yes. See. Don't move any of these ever. (In that way the child is sure to win the game and he proceeds to do just that. Then suddenly he sweeps all the draughts into a pile.) This will be a new game. Pile them all up. You pile those all up. Red are mine. The black are yours. Now we will have a battle. (The child moves his men and then he moves the therapist's men. He moves both sets of men, jumping them over one another.) He is a big man. This one. He is a giant. He can do anything in all the world. (He jumps over the therapist's men. He knocks some of them off the board.)

Therapist: Whoever he is, he certainly is powerful.

Child: He can do anything.

You see how the therapist does not attempt to rescue or direct the child's play, but reflects back what they see? This enables the child to express their anger and frustration at his father (Axline, 1969, p. 120).

References

Axline, V.M. (1969). *Play Therapy*. New York: Ballantine Books.

Bettelheim, B. (1975). *The Uses of Enchantment: The Meaning and Importance of Fairy Tales*. New York, Alfred Knopf.

Bradway, K. and McCoard, B. (2010). *Sandplay – Silent Workshop of the Psyche*. London, Routledge.

Chetwynd, T. (1982). *Dictionary of Symbols*. London: HarperCollins.

Hill, G.S. (1992). *Masculine and Feminine: The Natural Flow of Opposites in the Psyche*. London: Shambhala.

Dalley, T., Case, C., Schaverien, J., Weir, F., Halliday, D., Nowell Hall, P. and Waller, D. (1987). *Images in Art Therapy: New Developments in Theory and Practice*. London: Tavistock/Routledge.

Jung, C.J. (1958). *Psyche and Symbol*. New York: Doubleday.

Tressider, J. (2003). *10001 Symbols: The Illustrated Key to the World of Symbols*. London: Duncan Baird Publishers.

Turner, B.A. (2005). *The Handbook of Sandplay Therapy*. Cloverdale, CA: Temenos Press.

Chapter 7

Celebration

Introduction

I don't know many situations that aren't improved by cake! It plays a central role in most of my celebrations. Children never say no to some form of cake, which is why I asked PH to draw a picture of her most favourite cake.

The child is ready to recognise her achievement and to move forwards. A celebration is in order both on and off the page.

When a child's play therapy comes to an end, the final session has a celebratory theme. This is where we look at the progress they have made during their sessions. Sometimes this review takes the form of looking at the contents of the child's special box, the objects they have made – paintings, drawings, clay objects – all of which have special significance and represent a stage or moment in their journey, and other times they want to party! And part of this can involve not paying too much close attention to their box contents. Rarely have I had a child who didn't want to take their special box home, but sometimes they aren't ready to reflect so directly on their process during the final session. Parents tell me afterwards how the child showed them each object at home, which is the most important place for them to be shown and shared.

I always offer the party element to the child and invite them to choose something they would like to eat and drink. I set this out like a picnic on the floor, and this becomes the final shared moment. Some children find the ending especially hard and don't want to celebrate; for them the ending is another loss. It's important to recognise this aspect of the ending and to observe how they cope with the prospective separation from me. Some will be jubilant and others will be sad. All I can hope for is that during the sessions they have taken in enough to carry them through and beyond the separation. At its best I hope they will understand that they can tolerate the separation more resiliently.

DOI: 10.4324/9781003182009-9

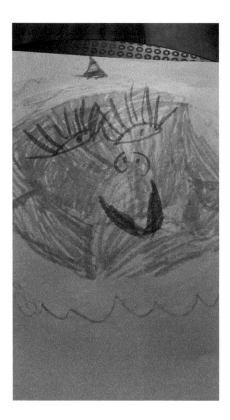

Figure 7.1 PH's unicorn cake.

A celebration can be offered at the completion of any stage in the hero's journey. It is simply a recognition of the completion of one stage and the readiness for the next part of the journey. In choosing to offer a celebration you are offering the child a moment of unconditional praise and acceptance. Equally, if you offer it and the child refuses, don't be upset by this or think you have done anything wrong. You haven't. The child isn't ready yet to acknowledge their own growth. Work with this. Allow them some space, and also offer them space to reflect with you on their progress. Don't just leave them hanging!

During the reflective stage, I'd like you to consider what question is left unanswered. Is there one or are there several? Go back to the start of the journey and refresh your memory about what the central quest was about. How far has the child travelled? What have they learned about themselves, their environment and their heroic quest?

The Helping Children Smile Again Reflective Practice

1. Does the child's story show signs of resilience?
2. What new strengths have emerged?
3. Does their journey show coping resources or channels of conflict?

4. Does their journey reveal developmental concerns and conflicts that belong to a young age or are not at all age appropriate?
5. Are the child's problems chronic or is the quest circular, so that a supportive approach may be the most suitable recommendation?

The cake image in this chapter was created by a young girl, PH. For her, cake represents the joyful and exciting aspects of a celebration. It's one of the resources she would take with her on her next journey. That's the other thing. Pay attention and review the symbols in the objects the child has created during their journey. These give you an opportunity to learn more about the child. PH has named her cake 'the unicorn cake'. A question I would ask is: 'Would you like to tell me more about the unicorn in your cake?' It's likely that knowing more about the unicorn would help me to understand more about what is important to PH – What role does the unicorn play in her life? What does the unicorn represent to her? What message does the unicorn carry for her? All of these 'discovery questions' could be incorporated into our celebration. You could physically provide some cake to be eaten during the celebration. You could 'bake' a cake as part of your celebration ceremony or draw one, there any number of ways you can expand on the resources the child has identified as being important, as she has done. Including these resources in the celebration affirms for the child that you have heard them and support them in their choices, both of which are very important for their self-esteem and confidence.

Chapter 8

Setting up a hero's journey storytelling group

There are some things working with a group can achieve that working with an individual cannot. Like dynamics. Working in a group setting holds up a mirror, and allows people to witness not only themselves through the others' eyes, but something that they had not seen before about other group members, who may reveal something about themselves they had not seen. If done well, a group dynamic is a solid practising ground to test out new theories and concepts. While it can make some feel vulnerable, it can also provide a safety net for experimentation which not only confronts but also comforts vulnerability. It's an opportunity to flex unused muscles and learn.

I always find it interesting to discover how each group has its own dynamic flavour. It's not unusual for participants to develop a group theme and personality. Each person is held within and by the group, which becomes an entity in itself.

Setting up a group is a particularly helpful way of introducing children to a new concept or way of seeing the world.

Below is the case study of a group I led in a primary school. This will give you a taster of how to use therapeutic play in a group format. Each child who took part in this group went on their own heroic journey. I have included notes about these individual journeys, and given a six-week group timetable of what to consider for each step of the journey.

Case study

This group case study describes the six directed play therapy sessions of a small group of children at the Malcolm Sargent Primary School, Lincolnshire, facilitated by Amanda Seyderhelm in 2015.

DOI: 10.4324/9781003182009-10

Group set-up

Small group

I elected to have groups of four children. This number allowed for the dynamics of small group communication to manifest, and helped each child to establish a strong self-concept.

Theme

A mission to space.

Focus

To promote building peer relationships.

In Egolf (2001, p. 12), Erikson says there is usually an individual or group that has a significant impact on development and self-concept. During the sixth year until the onset of puberty, the neighbours and school provide significant other groups. My case group were aged between 9 and 10 years, and, therefore, the focus of building peer relationships was an appropriate choice for their development.

Social behaviour of this age group is normally characterised by give and take, and more negotiation being possible in conflict situations (Geldard and Geldard, 2001, p. 40). The group provided the children with a safe space to struggle with and overcome some of these problematic behaviours.

Aims

To listen, accept one another and learn to work collaboratively.

Axline (1983, p. 25) argues that the group experience provides a realistic element because the child lives in the world with other children, and must consider the reaction of others and develop consideration for the feelings of other individuals.

It was hoped that by working in a group rather than individually, these four children would experience a sense of belonging, which would help them to develop positive feelings about themselves, address problem issues and engage in personal growth through working together to pursue a common goal with the aim of achieving a positive outcome for the whole group.

Type of group

A closed therapeutic group.

Planning

Location

All sessions took place in the play therapy room at the Malcolm Sargent Primary School on a Thursday at 2pm.

Child protection

I established a relationship with the school's Child Protection Officer, and understood the school's policy on child protection in the event of any disclosure being made in the group.

Health and Safety and Risk Assessment

The play therapy room had been risk assessed, and was near a toilet. The room itself was spacious, and suitably furnished to allow the planned activities to be carried out.

Confidentiality

A privacy notice was posted on the door, and all staff had been informed of what was happening and agreed not to interrupt the sessions. The play therapy room was situated some distance from the main classrooms, which ensured a degree of separateness from the main school areas. Symbolically, this enabled children to recognise that within the group there may be a different set of norms, particularly regarding their freedom of expression (Geldard and Geldard, 2001, p. 50).

Length of group sessions and overall duration

The group met for six non-consecutive weekly sessions each lasting 50 minutes.

Session work plan

Figure 8.6 shows my Mission to Space six-week group lesson plan.

Role and theoretical approach

My role was to facilitate the work plan during the group sessions, and to observe and influence group processes so that goals for both individual children and the group could be met. Geldard and Geldard say: 'Children in a democratically run group tend to be more productive as they feel included in group decision making' (2001, p. 100). My aim was to be creative and flexible and, as you will see, there were times when a consensus could not be reached, and my role then was to help the sub-groups become effective and productive.

Supervision

Twice-monthly supervision enabled me to process the strong transferences and counter-transferences, and to acknowledge when I was tempted to rescue group members from experiencing their own challenges and help them find their own solutions. By learning from this, I was able to hold the group with a lighter touch, and to facilitate this to develop in the way that it did.

Intake process and assessment

Intake process

The SENCO and I selected four children, two boys (JR and ZP aged 10 years) and two girls (IM and EP aged 9 years). Their assessment had taken into account their physical, emotional and psychological resources, and we agreed that this group would enable a balanced composition to be created. The children had similar needs regarding forming working peer relationships.

Assessment

The SENCO informed the parents about the purpose and assessment process of the group, and I met with the parents and teachers of all four children to obtain their consent, and complete Strengths and Difficulties Questionnaires (SDQs).

All the parents were supportive and encouraging about their children joining this group. Some parents raised anxieties concerning their child's emotional needs which I addressed in their end reviews.

The group programme

Egolf (2001, p.105) divided group development into four stages: Forming, Storming, Norming and Performing.

Session 1

Session topic: Set up.
  Stage of group development: getting started and forming the group contract.

Creating rapport in the circle
The weekly check-in ritual of 'welcome beads' was designed to draw the children into a circle formation and establish rapport. New research from the Sauder School of Business (2013) shows that seating arrangements can have a major impact on the way people think. People sitting in a circular formation are more likely to want to 'belong' to a group and are less prone to be antagonistic. Herman Miller's (2006) research shows that proximity in a circle formation may also help with collaboration and connectedness. We used the circle to contain discussions and debriefs. During the session, the circle changed shape as the children's process required them to step in and out of the circle. During times of anxiety, the children expressed their feelings through their body movements: ZP edged closer into the corner wall; JR stood with his hands in his pockets; IM pushed her back up against the wall; EP sat silently still with her legs crossed.

HTP drawings and the beginning of containment

The HTP projective assessment technique developed by John Buck was used weekly to assess the children's unconscious difficulties. I chose this form of assessment after learning that EP had difficulty speaking up in groups. Buck assumed that when the subject is drawing the children are projecting their inner world onto the page (Wikipedia, 2012). To form the circle boundary, I laid out four circular paper plates for their drawings. There was an atmosphere of intense concentration while the group drew. Initially they looked at one another's drawings, but by session 2 I felt more relaxed, and they drew silently. This was an instructive, if somewhat time-consuming exercise that helped them to start expressing and containing themselves.

Rather than handing out the session books, I placed them in a pile, and invited the children to choose their own coloured book. ZP immediately chose the pink book (it reminded him of spring flowers). IM chose orange because she liked Jaffa oranges, and EP chose red because it reminded her of her hamster's cage. JR took the remaining book.

After I'd I explained the contract rules, they wrote their individual names on the contract. I explained that the decisions were going to be made by them, and that my role was to help the group achieve its goals and to do this in ways which the group collectively chose.

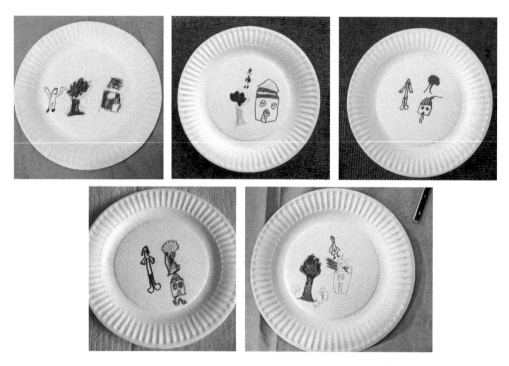

Figure 8.1–5 IM'S HTP drawings from five sessions of the Group Mission to Space. By session 5, the house is in proportion to the tree and child. The tree has flowers planted around it. The pink on the roof may suggest the release of stuck feelings.

Early group formation

The group started to form during a discussion about naming the planet. They wrote their planet names on paper, and decided they would like to stick the paper up on the wall next to their contract. This led to a discussion about secrecy and privacy, and they agreed that they wanted their list of planet names to be both secret and private. This opened up a discussion about the options for creating those conditions, and they agreed to tuck the paper behind their contract. ZP folded the page into a small size, and IM tucked the paper behind the contract, while ZP took sticky tape, and sealed one side of the contract page. JR was quiet. This meant that they could still access the list from the other open side.

ZP wanted to impose consequences on anyone who read or moved their list. Again we talked through some of those consequences, and they agreed to write the consequences down on the front of the folded list. This discussion was an early example of their eagerness to contribute ideas and form their own contract.

Session 2

Session topic: What does the planet look like?

Stage of group development: Forming.

In Stage 1, Forming, group members are concerned with orientation matters, finding and testing the boundaries (Egolf, 2001, p.102).

During this session, ZP and IM started asserting their voices and contributing ideas, and were successful in encouraging JR and EP to do the same. This was again evident when I asked who could remember the rules, and explain them to JR. Both IM and ZP said what happened in the room was a secret, and not to be talked about outside the room. I wondered what connotation the word 'secrecy' had for them. The parents of JR and ZP confirmed during end reviews that both boys had emphasised the importance of the rule of confidentiality, and not talked to them about the content of the sessions.

Recognising transference

I felt able to hold the group until they couldn't agree on a single planet name. This disagreement was a reflection of their lack of cohesion as a group, and one of the ways in which they remained uncovered. I wondered how to resolve this. Eventually, I realised that the resolution (or not) of their disagreement was as much part of their process and development as it was mine. So I asked them how they would like to resolve their disagreement. ZP and IM each took a leadership role by choosing two large sheets of paper and discussing whether they should Sellotape or glue these together. JR and EP stood silently beside them watching. I did not speak, and held this tension until ZP said out loud 'Do either of you have any suggestions yet?' This direct invitation moved JR further into the group, and he made some animals for the planet out of wool and pipe cleaners and stuck these onto the paper.

EP silently drew bridges between JR's animals. Within her silence, EP was holding herself and connecting with JR. This silent alliance between them continued throughout the group.

The check-out boundary

The circle check-out was a time for them to voice what they had, or hadn't, enjoyed about the session. ZP said he had enjoyed the whole session and the way they had worked together. JR said he liked the way no-one had said 'No', and everyone had taken on board other people's ideas. EP said she enjoyed being able to create her idea. I reflected on how children tell you their truth when invited to do so and given a safe space to be heard.

Session 3

Session topic: What kind of aliens will be on the planet?
   Stage of group development: Storming.
   Storming refers to the conflict phase of group development. Conflict refers to the anxiety generated when a choice between or among alternatives must be made (Egolf, 2001, p. 115).

Learning to express and contain discomfort

This session marked a turning point for IM in her processing, and allowed the group to dramatically express and contain their feelings through puppetry.

   IM was unhappy about attending the session because she didn't want to miss her choir practice, and was crying when I collected her from the hall. The other three children were with me. Remembering how my Diploma Course Director had encouraged me to take my storming feelings into the group, I encouraged IM to do the same. She reluctantly agreed. I was nervous about how to contain her misery, and held this until we sat in the circle and had completed the check-in ritual. I explained how sometimes it could be difficult when someone was missing from a group, and I asked them how they would feel if they were not present. ZP said that he would miss out on some learning, JR reassured IM by saying that she had attended all the other choir practices and was not missing out on any new songs.

   IM was not consoled. Tears rolled down her cheeks as she drew her HTP drawing. We looked into one another's eyes, and I could feel her cry to be rescued, and noticed how much I wanted to 'make it better' for her. At that moment I realised how doing so would not only have drawn my attention away from the other group members but would also have denied her the experience of sitting with her own feelings of discomfort. Instead I gave her the space to sit silently with her own feelings, and she eventually rejoined the group. During this time the other children looked over at IM, and continued to draw. The group boundary had remained intact, and allowed IM to sit still. Aware of her bereavement, I followed up with her teacher after the session.

Creating puppet characters, and finding the unfrozen voice

Aronoff (1995, p. 1), who uses puppets in her work with children in hospital, refers to the way puppets 'speak' for the 'frozen voice' of the child. The client-puppeteer, whether in individual therapy or group work, can be seen as director, actor and audience simultaneously.

Therapeutic Puppetry (2005) argues that puppetry's advantage over other methods is its safe indirectness: one can rehearse for 'real' life. You can play, get input from the therapist or the group and replay differently.

I had chosen puppets to give the children a medium through which to claim their projective parts. As a result of doing so, they would be ready to integrate a split-off role (Jennings, 1999, p. 107). Angry puppet play followed. Led by IM, they enacted a puppet play that saw their unfrozen voices speaking through duels, fighting over who was right, with instances of one puppet hitting another. Eventually this was resolved in the puppet play, and I wonder if this enabled them to enact their own issues in role and then move towards integration. Proof of this was the feedback from their teachers, who reported an improvement in anger management.

Speaking for the National Association for the Education of Young People (NAEYC) (2001), Gussin Paley said:

> Think dramatically. Get in the habit of thinking of yourself and the children as partners in an acting company. Once we learn to imagine ourselves as characters in a story, a particular set of events expands in all directions. We find ourselves being kinder and more respectful to one another because our options have grown in intimacy, humour, and literary flavour.
>
> (NAEYC, 2001)

I reflected on the placement of the puppets on the planet, and how these changed positions perhaps indicated the internal shifts the children were making: EP's character was on the outer edges of the planet, and she moved it closer to the middle. IM moved her character nearer to EP's. Both JR and ZP placed their characters alongside each other. I wondered in what ways the puppets' positions might also be a reflection of the children's identification with one another.

Through enacting dramatic puppet stories, the children had expanded the energy of the group, and perhaps some of their feelings aroused by that discussion, and the group dynamics.

Session 4

Session topic: Prepare to journey in the space rocket.

   Stage of group development: Norming.

During the Norming stage of group development, conflicts are resolved, new standards and roles emerge and members can communicate more freely. The group shifts from the 'I' and becomes 'We' (Egolf, 2001, p. 129).

Learning to reach a consensus

The group learned the value of talking to reach a consensus before taking any action, and reached a new level of cohesiveness, following the shared emotional experience of session 3.

   The task was to build their space rocket. They stood around looking at one another unsure how to start. Then they started throwing out ideas about building the space rocket. I asked them what they needed to do first and immediately ZP said: 'Design the rocket!' This suggestion got drowned out by IM who wanted her ideas to be chosen. I acknowledged them all, reminded them about their time limit, and suggested they start building. They ripped open boxes, glued them together and decorated them. ZP and JR worked together, and EP and IM worked individually, and separately from the others. Near the end of the time for building, I asked them to pause and review their progress. At this point it became apparent that three of them (ZP, JR and IM) had all built the front part of the rocket!

EP was the only one who had created a top part. When they realised they had two front ends, I saw the realisation dawn on their faces and asked them how they could have avoided making two front ends. They all said: 'Talk to one another.' This then opened the door for them to join all the parts together and form one rocket, which was preparation for them to tell their sandtray story.

Session 5

Session task: Make space outfits and take the journey to the sand planet.

   Stage of group development: Performing.

   During the Performing stage of development, the successful group settles down and begins to do what it is supposed to do: complete its task (Egolf, 2001, p. 140).

Telling the sandtray story

By this stage I was feeling pressurised to complete the group's tasks in six sessions because I was struggling to hold all four processes within the six-week timeframe. A factor which contributed to my struggle was the weekly HTP drawing. By doing this, the children went into a deeper process and everything took longer. On reflection, I may have saved time by using the Blob Man as a check-in tool. However, in supervision, I learnt to maintain stronger time boundaries around each task and not to devote too much time to any one child.

   This challenge was reflected in the space outfit making, where IM attempted more storming. JR decisively chose to wear a black robe which he decorated with space lettering. He was unequivocal about his choice, demonstrating his renewed confidence. IM and ZP decided to draw straws for an outfit. IM looked miserable after losing the draw, and took some time before she was willing to try on something else. I felt uncomfortable about IM's misery over being unable to have what she wanted, but contained my anxiety while she chose something else to wear. This showed me the strength of the transference. IM's demand for attention was in sharp contrast to EP's contained silence throughout all the sessions, which provided me with a personal learning opportunity.

   When they were dressed in their outfits, they carried their rocket into the sandtray and made their sandtray story. Now more comfortable in their roles, they all contributed enthusiastically to the sandtray story, taking it in turns to add miniatures to the sand and talking about their characters as they placed them in the sandtray.

Gradually the sandtray filled up, and they sat around the tray telling the story, although JR stood up. There was an atmosphere of collaboration between them. Towards the end of the session, they picked up their puppet characters and engaged them in conversation. They let off steam, laughing and joking, relieved, perhaps, to have made their journey.

Session 6

Session topic: Homecoming and separation.

Stage of group development: Celebrating and reflecting.

After the medal-making, which involved sharing of resources and a ceremonial photograph, we returned to the circle for a debrief.

There were mixed feelings about the group ending. Neither of the boys wanted the group to end, and said they had enjoyed using their imaginations and that it had helped them to make friends outside the group. This was brilliant to hear because the group was set up to help build peer relationships. Both girls were less enthusiastic. EP said she had enjoyed everything about the group but would miss nothing! IM said she had enjoyed missing her lessons!

End reviews with parents and teachers

All parents said their children made some progress while being in the group, and generally they had seen improvements in them being able to hold and contain their feelings. Teachers reported back to me on how the hoped-for outcomes had been achieved: JR was much better at group work and playing with his peers at break time, and was less isolated in class. ZP had an improved awareness of social cues, understood the rules of friendship and was controlling his temper. IM had shown a big improvement in her temper control and ability to tolerate someone else's point of view. EP was slowly coming out of her shell.

Conclusion

Overall the children achieved the aims of the group. They listened to each other's points of view and learned to accept the differences, value and challenges involved in working collaboratively.

The boys in particular found a sense of belonging in the group, through being fully heard and accepted as they are. This was a new experience for both boys, and one which they took back into their classrooms and homes. IM learned to sit with her difficult feelings and to contain them. EP overcame her fears of being in a group by working with the others in pursuit of a common goal.

They all understood the importance of sharing a task, helping one another and recognising when they needed to plan out loud rather than by themselves. I facilitated change by providing the children with an opportunity to learn skills involved in giving and receiving feedback. By providing feedback to help others, the children in this group learned strategies to help themselves.

According to Taylor (2003, p. 99), the bond a group needs in order to establish itself can be thought of as: 'the minimum level of commitment required to function effectively enough to accomplish the tasks it is set up to do'.

This group achieved the minimum level, and was able to function as a group. Each one surrendered some of their 'preciousness' to do what they like in favour of making a contribution to the group. We worked through their concerns around loss of individuality, and I facilitated this by encouraging them to talk about their concerns in the group so that the less vocal members (JR and EP) could feel included.

Theoretical background

When setting up a group it is important to be clear about the *theoretical orientation* and the type of group you are running to be able to facilitate change and learning in children.

Type of group
We were running a closed, topic-focused and time-limited group, where the members all joined simultaneously and had similar needs and compatible developmental levels. The group ran for a predetermined number of sessions. Our topic was to help children build peer relationships by planning a mission into space and we followed Play Therapy UK's (PTUK's) assessment rules.

The *leadership style* and structure of our group was based on using the Play Therapy Dimensions Model which uses a combination of a behavioural (directive) and experiential, person-centred (non-directive) approach. This means we were interactively directing and orchestrating the work of the group by setting weekly activities and creative experiments drawn from the Play Therapy Kit to help the children experience and understand the meaning of their behaviours, as well as reflecting and commenting on their interactions and play.

Integrating elements
We recognised that if issues of transference and counter-transference needed to be addressed, it may be useful for us to introduce solution-focused problem solving from a post-modern approach, where we would help the child to form particular goals by using specific questioning techniques.

Perspective
Patricia Hasbach, a psychotherapist and coauthor with Peter Kahn of the book *Ecopsychology: Science, Totems, and the Technological Species* (2012), uses the analogy of a camera to explain the connection between psychology and nature: by opening the lens wider, you are able to shift the focus from the individual to the wider natural world.

In the early days of clinical psychology, thanks in part to Freud, who believed that nature 'destroys us – coldly, cruelly, relentlessly' (Freud, 1917/2005), the focus of the field was narrow, taking in just the contents of one person's mind, ego, super-ego and id.

Subsequently, psychology broadened its scope to look at relationships between people, then to interactions in whole families, then to society at large. Now the lens is opening wider still to include the natural world.

Types of theoretical approach used by group leaders to produce change

It is important for group leaders to have a clear understanding of which approach they should use.

Psychoanalytic approach: make unconscious motives conscious.
The child changes old patterns by working through the transference distortions.
Group approach: therapist treats the group as a whole and assists the group to look for latent themes underlying the manifest behaviour.
Experiential approach: client-centred therapy.
Rogers and Gestalt utilise the phenomenological method – taking the client's ongoing awareness of their own experience as the primary datum for therapy.
Defines the facilitation of experiencing as the key therapeutic task – discovery orientated. Seeks to further the client's potential for growth, self-determination and choice. New and/or raised awareness and the generation of new meaning are the basis of change.
Post-modern approach: clients behave like scientists, formulating hypotheses to explain life's experiences, testing and revising them as new experiences are encountered.
Solution-focused therapy approach: therapist helps the client form specific goals.
Narrative therapy approach: clients find meaning by organising their experiences and external events into stories. As clients tell their stories, the therapist helps them both to discover that these stories are social constructions that are not fixed and to realise that other stories may be more suitable.
Cognitive/behaviour approach: helps children modify their attitudes, beliefs and constructs about life and change their behaviours. Emphasises the role of thinking, questioning, deciding, doing and re-deciding. Psycho-educational as it emphasises therapy as a learning process.
Behaviour therapy approach: focuses on current overt behaviour and assumes behaviour is learnt through reinforcement and imitation. Client encouraged to set goals and experiment with new behaviours. Therapist is active and directive but ignores underlying emotional and psychological issues.
Developmental approach: Piaget (1980) and Kohlberg (1984).
Based on the concept of children acquiring particular behaviours and skills at various stages in their development. This leads to group leaders having expectations about change and outcomes consistent with the group members' levels of development. To bring about change, leaders need to provide opportunities that progressively extend the child's cognitive, social, emotional and moral development.

Figure 8.6 Lesson plan.

Week	Session topic	Session goal	Session method	Check-in	Activities	Ending	Resources
1	**Set up**	Explain & sign Contract	Group	*Beads on a string; Tree House Person	All members to sign group contract	Therapist to add session photo; decorate star for session book; All hold bead cord and say **1 good thing	Beads, space workbook x 4, roll of paper, paper plates, pens, crayons, scissors, glue
2	**What does the planet look like?**	Forming	Group	Beads on a string; Tree House Person	Design planet on paper	As above	Beads, workbooks, different paper sizes and colours, pens, crayons, string, wool, scissors, glue
3	**What kind of aliens will be on the planet?**	Storming	Individually & in pairs	Beads on a string; Tree House Person	Make alien puppet characters	As above	Beads, workbooks, wooden spoons, wool, wire, googly eyes, pens, crayons, glue, scissors
4	**Prepare to journey**	Norming	As part of team	Beads on a string; Tree House Person	Build space rocket using junk modelling	As above	Beads, workbooks, card boxes, pens, string, wool, paper, glue, scissors

| 5 | Take the journey | Performing | Individually and group | Beads on a string; Tree House Person | Make space outfits & land on the sand planet | As above | Beads, workbooks, shirts, space outfits, foil, sandtray, miniatures. |
| 6 | Homecoming & separation | Celebrating | Individually and group | Beads on a string; Tree House Person | Create medals & review books | As above | Beads, workbooks, card, string, pens, crayons, glue, scissors |

*Welcome ritual: beads on a string. We moved around the circle and said hello, my name is and one thing we had enjoyed about our day. Designed to form a connection.

**Saying one good thing: children used this time to share both good and difficult experiences during their day, and their session. It was used to set an upbeat tone for the beginning of the session, and to close the session with something they had learned.

References

Aronoff, M. (1995). 'Puppets Go Hand in Hand with Loss'. In Children in Scotland Conference Report, *Working with Loss.*

Astell-Burt, C. (2001). *I am the Story, the Art of Puppetry in Education and Therapy.* London: Souvenir Press.

Axline, V. M. (1983). *Play Therapy.* New York: Ballantine Books.

Egolf, D.B. (2001). *Forming, Storming, Norming, Performing.* Lincoln, NE: Writer's Club Press.

Erikson, E.H. (1995). *Childhood and Society.* London: Vintage.

Freud, S. (1917/2005). *On Murder, Mourning and Melancholia.* London: Penguin Books.

Geldard, K. and Geldard, D. (2001).*Working with Children in Groups: A Handbook for Counsellors, Educators, and Community Workers.* Basingstoke: Palgrave.

Gibbs, J.C. (2019). *Moral Development and Reality. Beyond the Theories of Kohlberg, Hoffman, and Haidt.* Oxford: Oxford University Press.

Jennings, S. (1999). *Dramatherapy: Theory and Practice 2.* London: Routledge.

Khan, P.H. and Hasbach, P.H. (eds) (2012). *Ecopsychology: Science, Totems, and the Technological Species.* Cambridge, MA: MIT Press.

Miller, H. (2006). 'Rethinking the classroom: spaces designed for active and engaged learning and teaching' (Online). Available at: www.hermanmiller.com/research/solution-essays/rethinking-the-classroom.html. Accessed 6 August 2015.

National Association for the Education of Young People (NAEYC) (2001). 'A conversation with Vivian Gussin Paley' (Online). Available at: www.naeyc.org/content/conversation-vivian-gussin-paley. Accessed 27 July 2015.

Piaget, J. (1980). *Play, Dreams, and Imitation in Childhood.* Hassell Street Press.

Sauder School of Business (2013). 'Want consensus in the boardroom? Get round a table' (Online). Available at: www.sauder.ubc.ca/News/2013. Accessed 27 July 2015.

Taylor, B. (2003). *Forging the Future Together: Human Relations in the 21st Century.* Yorkshire: Oasis Press.

Therapeutic Puppetry (2005). 'Therapeutic puppetry – empowering, transforming, healing' (Online). Available at: www.therapeuticpuppetry.com. Accessed 28 July 2015.

Wikipedia (2012). 'House-Tree-Person Test' (Online). Available at: https://en.wikipedia.org/wiki/House-Tree-Person_test. Accessed 17 August 2015.

Chapter 9

When to seek further support

The referral process to external intervention services has never been more complex. Waiting lists for CAMHS support have doubled since I published my first book in 2020. Wherever possible, I recommend schools find creative ways to offer further support within the school environment in order to avoid exclusions. This is much easier for children to accommodate than having to leave school to attend an appointment. It's why I believe every school should have at least one qualified counsellor or play therapist on permanent staff. Investing in training for these staff is going to make the experience of 'further support' more cohesive for all concerned.

I offer CPD training in schools on how to shift the culture towards using a therapeutic approach to help children express their feelings. You can find details about these trainings on www.helpingchildrensmileagain.com.

Let's remember that children are negotiating invisible endings and transitions throughout their day, and when they are coping with these in addition to sensory overload, SEN and ACES, the last thing they need is to have to leave the school for 'further support' only to re-enter again an hour later. It can often undo all the good they receive during their therapy sessions.

Let's consider just some of these invisible endings and transitions:

- Leaving the classroom
- Re-entering the classroom
- Ending a conversation
- Starting a conversation
- Ending some work
- Starting a new piece of work
- Starting lunch break
- Ending lunch break
- Starting playtime
- Ending playtime

DOI: 10.4324/9781003182009-11

When children are on sensory overload endings and transitions are especially difficult to cope with, so they will need you to stand and be alongside them during these times. Listen first. Reflect back what you see and hear, and help them to name their feelings.

By doing these things, you are making their struggles bearable and their feelings visible.

Be their hero.

Appendices

The red flag list

A person's behaviour is a signal that something is either wrong or right. Behaviour is the child's way of waving a red flag in order to get your attention. Be aware of the behaviours listed below in the classroom because the child may be indicating that they are struggling with loss and change. Don't be too quick to raise the ADHD flag! I see this a lot in schools and it's easy to make this assumption when the behavior traits are similar, but this does not necessarily mean the child has ADHD. First check that the child has not experienced some type of loss or change.

Always focus on what is driving the behaviour rather than the behaviour itself because that is where you start to build a connection with the child. This is why punishment/reward doesn't work. It may have the effect of stopping the behaviour but it will not create a meaningful or lasting change in the child who has empathy and compassion at its heart.

- Deterioration in focus and concentration.
- Being fidgety and unable to settle down to complete a task.
- Jumping from one thing to another.
- A sudden change in mood.
- Angry outbursts.
- Being unusually clingy.
- Tiredness – yawning or falling asleep in class.

APPENDIX 2

The meaning of colours

- *White* – healing light, spiritual guidance, direction to the right path.
- *Red* – courage, energy, ability to take action, love, passion.
- *Yellow* – power of the mind, mental creativity, confidence.
- *Orange* – ability to change your luck and take control of your situation, energy.

- *Blue* – harmony, understanding, spiritual journey, loyalty, wisdom, protection.
- *Green* – balance, practical creativity, growth, health.
- *Brown* – defence, protection, counteraction, banishing evil.
- *Indigo* – discovering past lives, sorting karmic problems, balancing karma, breaking repeating karmic patterns.
- *Purple* – most powerful meditation colour, psychic and spiritual growth, healing, power, independence.

APPENDIX 3

Glossary

Acting out Exhibiting destructive behaviour that discharges the energy of your emotions but results in negative consequences for yourself and others.

Adult Self The responsible part of yourself that governs your daily life.

Boundaries Personal boundaries are guidelines, rules or limits that a person creates to identify reasonable, safe and permissible ways for other people to behave towards them and how they will respond when someone passes those limits.

Centre of your being For most people this is the place in your body at the very bottom of your diaphragm. It is where your breath leads you when you inhale deeply.

Codependency An inability to fulfill your primary needs because your focus is always on meeting the needs of the person upon whom you are emotionally or financially dependent; ordinarily this is due to patterns of behaviour learned in childhood to ensure survival which result in low self-esteem.

Developmental stages Predictable stages of emotional growth that occur in the natural progression from birth to adulthood. Each stage has specific tasks that need to be mastered if this progression is to take place successfully.

Generalised grief Grief that extends beyond your personal experience; feeling the pain of others that is similar or the same as your own.

Guided imagery A structured imaginative fantasy the purpose of which is to aid your internal exploration. You create images or scenes in your mind's eye and then relate to those images, directing them much as you would a play. Guided imagery does not always elicit visual responses; sometimes the scenes are evoked by recalling certain smells or tastes or by hearing sounds of the scene being described.

Higher power For some it is the image of a wise old being; for others it may be a sphere of light, a guardian angel or a spirit guide. For some it is experienced as part of the Self; for others it will be something outside the Self. The image may be based on religious beliefs, appearing in the form of Jesus, the Buddha, Mohammed or a guru; others may experience it as an abstract symbol of a Higher Self such as a cross or a mandala, or the intuitive or spiritual part of Self within you. Some may picture it as an aspect of nature, or a group to which one belongs.

Higher Self The spiritual dimension of Self.

Inherited grief Unresolved grief that is passed on from generation to generation until someone finally breaks the cycle and resolves the feelings of loss.

Inner child Small voices inside that carry childhood feelings.

Internal support group Supportive characters, real or imagined, that you bring into your guided imagery to support your exploration.

Journal   Writing that is used for personal reflections about your emotional and spiritual journey.

Mind's eye   Your imagination; what you see in your head when you close your eyes and play imaginative games.

Processing   Word used to describe the act of identifying, expressing and releasing feelings.

Protective light   A healing light connected with your Higher Power that you call on imaginatively to aid your internal explorations; a metaphor for the healing power of the universal spirit.

Recovery   The process of learning how to break addictive behaviour patterns and live with feelings non-addictively.

Ritual   A ceremony performed for the purpose of celebrating the completion of a phase of your internal work or to provide a tangible way of releasing pain.

Self-esteem   Describes your level of self-worth; how you feel about yourself. These feelings are generally based on how you were treated as a child. If you were treated with respect and you received love, you will have high self-esteem. If you were neglected, abused or abandoned, you will have low self-esteem and not feel very worthy.

Support system   Friends, family and others who believe in and encourage your personal growth.

APPENDIX 4

Story Template in 6 boxes

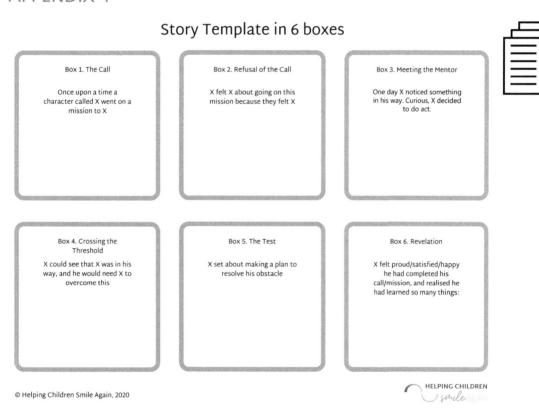

© Helping Children Smile Again, 2020

HELPING CHILDREN
smile again

Figure A.4 Template of a hero's story in six boxes.

APPENDIX 5

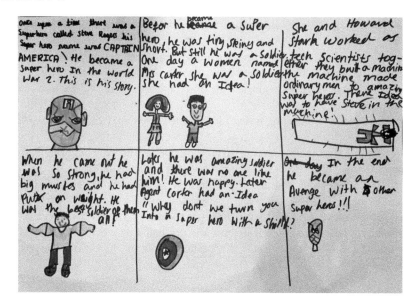

Figure A.5 Example of completed 6 box story template by a child at Great Ormond Street Hospital for Children.

APPENDIX 6

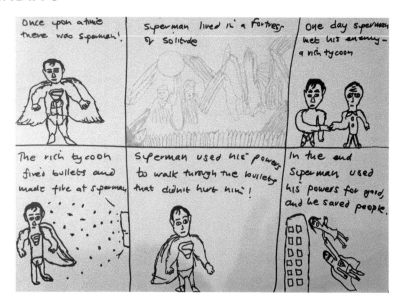

Figure A.6 Example of completed 6 box story template by a child at Great Ormond Street Hospital for Children.

APPENDIX 7

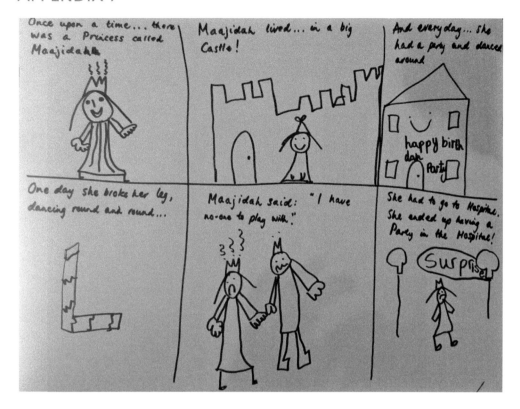

Figure A.7 Example of completed 6 box story template by a child at Great Ormond Street Hospital for Children.

APPENDIX 8

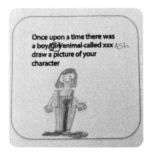
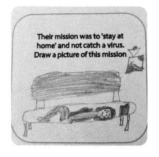
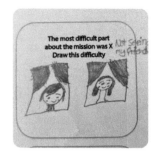
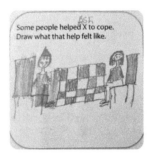
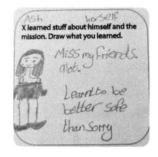
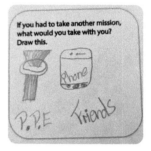

Figure A.8 Title: 'Better Safe than Sorry', completed 6 box story by O, an 8-year-old boy during lockdown. O's chosen resource is a torch, in box 6, which he would want to take with him in the event of another pandemic. This shows remarkable insight and proves that when a child is telling their story within the safe distance of metaphor, they show you their feelings. By decoding the messages within the story, we learn more about the child's needs. In this case, perhaps a need for certainty. The torch can become a talking point through which you can explore more about the child's need, and decide how to meet it.

APPENDIX 9

How to construct a therapeutic story using the hero's journey framework

Here is a story called 'Tilly Tea Pot' which appeared in *Helping Children Cope with Loss and Change*. I have deconstructed this for you so that you can see the sequence of writing a therapeutic story using the hero's journey framework. If you have a child who is not responding to other interventions, you could try using this framework to write a simple story to use with them.

Identify the emotional problem or issue

The child feels isolated from their classmates because they are the only mixed-race child at school.

Set a therapeutic objective – what would you like to change?

The objective is to enable the child to feel at ease and engaged. They should recognise that being different also means being unique.

Think of a strategy to achieve the change

The child meets people who object to them being treated differently. This advocacy on their behalf enables the child to feel included in the group and to use their voice to own their uniqueness.

Base the story on a metaphorical conflict in terms that the child can relate to – a character, a place, a plot grappling with the same emotional problem as the child. What similar stories or real-life experiences could be used?

The client is the only teapot made in a pottery factory that is put to one side because it has a crinkly spout.

Start constructing the story by thinking out the ending in outline

When the teapot hears the other pots standing up for her she realises that she's not alone and this gives her confidence to notice the differences between herself and the others and the things that make her and them unique. The result is that the client stops feeling isolated because she feels connected to the group of pots and is clear about her role and contribution to the teaset.

Write the start – set the scene

Tilly is a teapot. She has been made in a factory called Pots R Us that specialises in making teasets. The factory specifications are rigid and don't make allowances for any differences, all teapots have to look the same. But Tilly comes out of The Kiln with a crinkly spout instead of a straight one, and she therefore cannot be included in the teaset because she is different from her fellow teapots. This has never happened at the factory before, and no-one, including The Kiln, knows what to do. Seeing Tilly standing alone on a table puzzles the other pots. They don't know what to say to Tilly, and this leaves Tilly feeling isolated and lonely sitting on the table by herself. She wonders why she isn't included with the other pots.

Reach a metaphorical crisis

Tilly sits by herself on the table watching the pots being painted: some are given dots, others stripes, and she notices that she isn't being given either. She does notice that she is the only pot with a crinkly spout, and she wonders if that is why she has been excluded. This makes her feel sad. The sugar bowls and teapots are rattling their lids, and she thinks they are poking fun at her, and this makes her doubly sad. Instead of joining in she sits very still. She wants to shout at them and tell them that she's just like them really, but they are making so much noise she's afraid they won't hear her.

When The Box marches in with his lid open carrying a big roll of Sellotape in his arms Tilly's worst fears look as if they will come true. Tilly knows that The Box is getting ready to pack all the pots up into a teaset and send them off to a customer who has bought them! The prospect of the pots leaving Tilly all by herself creates a hush in the factory as the lids stop rattling. The cream jug and the sugar bowl notice that Tilly is alone. They both move out of their huddle and stand in a line facing Tilly. Tilly moves to the edge of her table and stares at them, a lone tear slides down her spout.

Construct the shift, the change of direction, using parallel learning situations – use a bridge section to avoid moving too quickly

Tilly catches the eye of Billy, the milk jug. Billy is slowly lifting his spout to wave at Tilly. Tilly wrinkles her crinkles in a slow smile. When Billy realises that Tilly wants to be friends with the other pots, and she's not sitting alone because she doesn't like them, he moves to the edge of the table and speaks out in Tilly's defence. He challenges Mr Conveyer Belt and tells him that if Tilly isn't part of their teaset and coming with them in the packing then they have no business calling the factory Pots R Us. Billy thought they were a team.

Billy is the leader of the pot gang, and when he speaks out in Tilly's defence all the other pots listen to him.

The Kiln hears the uproar and opens his door to find out what the noise is about.

He's not used to being questioned about his power to mould and manufacture pots. He has a recipe to follow, a quota to fill, that's all he cares about. But Billy stands up to him and tells him that the pots are upset that Tilly won't be joining their teaset. They are curious about Tilly's crinkles, and wonder why they don't have any.

Show the journey from crisis to positive solution and a new sense of identification

Tilly is surprised and delighted by Billy's advocacy, and the fact that the other pots really do want her to join their teaset. This feeling of empathy encourages her to look more closely at herself and at her fellow pots. As she examines both she sees that not all their stripes and dots are the same as she had originally assumed. When she re-examines her own crinkles she realises that she has more in common with her fellow pots than she thought. She notices the occasional dot in amongst her crinkles. This recognition of similarity makes her feel brave and excited about being at the beginning rather than the end of an adventure. Tilly suddenly moves closer to the edge of the table and finds the voice that she has been so nervous and scared of using. She claims her own identity as a crinkly teapot and announces that crinkles mean that she can pour in several directions and not just one! This announcement makes the other pots stand up proudly and say who they are – pots with wild stripes, lids with dazzling dots.

The Kiln is shocked by this show of collective team spirit, and for the first time marvels that the pots don't mind being different! What he thought were imperfections are actually marks of uniqueness. He apologises to the pots and tells them that from now on he will change his control panel setting from 'different' to 'unique'.

End the story with a celebration and sense of community

The Kiln instructs The Box to carry Tilly from her lonely table to join the other pots. But Tilly stops him. She raises her crinkly spout and says that she wants to make that journey by herself. As she says this she takes a small step and joints the pots on their table. As she steps over the gap she notices that the gap between the two tables is tiny and not as wide and cavernous as she had originally thought it was.

Tilly joins up the dots with the stripes and together they make a huge and colourful zigzag that dances around the shed. The Kiln turns on his lights and illuminates the factory shed with warm light and the whole teaset assembles on a blanket to enjoy their own special tea party.

APPENDIX 10

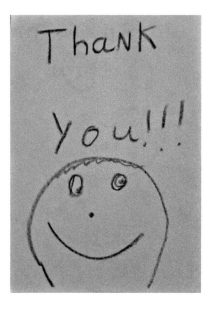

Figure A.10 Drawing completed by a child during their final session.

FINAL NOTE

Every person who has lived through the period 2020–2022 has their own heroic story to tell about the journey they have taken to cope and survive. That journey has been harder for some than others. We haven't all been in the same boat. We have all had to find our own torches to highlight our creative processes. Not all of our stories have been resolved, we are all at different points in our quest, but I hope that this book has given you a map to use to start your journey. To begin the dig. To know how to recognise your guide when they show up, and what to do when you hit obstacles. If this book has triggered you to review your own heroic journey, I want to encourage you to take your time to reflect on that. Go easy on yourself. There is no perfect time to start this. Trust yourself. Listen to your intuition. Let this guide you, and use the exercises in this book to light your path towards the resolution of your quest.

Bibliography

Academy of Play and Child Psychotherapy (APAC) (2014). Diploma in *Play Therapy Course*. Uckfield, East Sussex: APAC.

Allan, J. (1988). *Inscapes of the Child's World: Jungian Counseling in Schools and Clinics*. Dallas, TX: Spring Publications.

Aronoff, M. (1995). 'Puppets Go Hand in Hand with Loss'. In Children in Scotland Conference Report, *Working with Loss*.

Astell-Burt, C. (2001). *I am the Story, the Art of Puppetry in Education and Therapy*. London: Souvenir Press.

Axline, V. (1964). *DIBS In Search of Self*. Middlesex: Penguin Books.

Axline, V. (1969). *Play Therapy*. New York: Ballantine Books.

Barnardo's. (2020). 'New term, new challenges, new opportunities. Putting children's mental health at the heart of education'. August. Barnardo's Northern Ireland. Available at: https://www.barnardos.org.uk/sites/default/files/uploads/BarnardosNI-ChildrensMentalHealthAtTheHeartOfEducation.pdf[SC1] Challenges, New Opportunities.

Bettelheim, B. (1975). *The Uses of Enchantment: The Meaning and Importance of Fairy Tales*. New York: Alfred Knopf.

Binswinger, L. (1946). 'The existential analysis school of thought'. In R. May et al. (eds) *Existence*. New York: Basic Books.

Bowlby, J. (1998). *Attachment and Loss, Vol. 3: Loss: Sadness and Depression*. London: Pimlico.

Bradway, K. and McCoard, B. (2010). *Sandplay – Silent Workshop of the Psyche*. London, Routledge.

Brown, F. and Patte, M. (2013). *Rethinking Children's Play*. London: Bloomsbury.

Buck, J.N. (1948). 'The H-T-P', *Journal of Clinical Psychology*, 4, 151–159.

Bunce, M. and Rickards, A. (2004). 'Working with bereaved children: A guide. The Children's Legal Centre'. Available at: www1.essex.ac.uk/armedcon/unit/project/wwbc_guide/index.html.

Campbell, J. (2008). *The Hero with a Thousand Faces*. Novato, CA: New World Library.

Cantor, M.D. (2007). *The Use of Storytelling in Therapy with Children*. Northampton, MA: Smith College School for Social Work.

Chetwynd, T. (1982). *Dictionary of Symbols*. London: HarperCollins.

Bollas, C. (1987). *The Shadow of the Object, Psychoanalysis of the unthought known*. London: Free Association Books.

Combs, G. and Freedman, J. (1990). *Symbol, Story and Ceremony: Using Metaphor in Individual and Family Therapy*. New York: W.W. Norton & Company, Inc.

Dalley, T., Case, C., Schaverien, J., Weir, F., Halliday, D., Nowell Hall, P. and Waller, D. (1987). *Images in Art Therapy: New Developments in Theory and Practice*. London: Tavistock/Routledge.

Egolf, D.B. (2001). *Forming, Storming, Norming, Performing*. Lincoln, NE: Writer's Club Press.

Ellis, J., Dowrick, C. and Lloyd-Williams, M. (2013). 'The long-term impact of early parental death: lessons from a narrative study', *Journal of the Royal Society of Medicine*, 106(2), 57–67.

Erikson, E.H. (1995). *Childhood and Society*. London: Vintage.

Freud, S. (1917/2005). *On Murder, Mourning and Melancholia*. London: Penguin Books.

Furman, E. (1974). *A Child's Parent Dies: Studies in Childhood Bereavement*. New Haven, CT: Yale University Press.

Furth, G.M. (1988). *The Secret World of Drawings: A Jungian Approach to Healing through Art*. Toronto: Inner City Books.

Geldard, K. and Geldard, D. (2001).*Working with Children in Groups: A Handbook for Counsellors, Educators, and Community Workers*. Basingstoke: Palgrave.

Gersie, A. (1992). *Storymaking in Bereavement: Dragons Fight in the Meadow*. London: Jessica Kingsley Publishers.

Gibbs, J.C. (2019). *Moral Development and Reality. Beyond the Theories of Kohlberg, Hoffman, and Haidt*. Oxford: Oxford University Press.

Gibson, L.C. (2015). *Adult Children of Emotionally Immature Parents: How to Heal from Distant, Rejecting, or Self-involved Parents*. Oakland, CA: New Harbinger Publications.

Griffiths, A. and Denton, T. (2015). *The Treehouse Series*. London: Macmillan Children's Books.

Halprin, D. (2003). *The Expressive Body in Life, Art and Therapy: Working with Movement, Metaphor and Meaning*. London: Jessica Kingsley Publishers.

Hamilton, N. (1985). 'The alchemical process of transformation' (Online). Available at: www.sufismus.ch/assets/files/omega_dream/alchemy_e.pdf. Accessed 15 August 2015.

Hill, G.S. (1992). *Masculine and Feminine: The Natural Flow of Opposites in the Psyche*. London: Shambhala.

Hillman, J. (1997). *Suicide and the Soul*. Woodstock, CT: Spring Publications.

Hospice Education Institute (n.d.). 'Family therapy'. Available at: https://www.hospiceuk.org/what-we-offer/;publications. Accessed 17 May 2022.

Jennings, S. (1999). *Dramatherapy: Theory and Practice 2*. London: Routledge.

Johnson, R.A. (2008). *Inner Gold: Understanding Psychological Projection*. Ashville, NC: Koa Books.

Jung, C.J. (1958). *Psyche and Symbol*. New York: Doubleday

Jung, C.J. (1990). *The Archetypes and the Collective Unconscious*. London: Routledge.

Jung, C.J. (2014). 'Jung and alchemy' (Online). Available at: www.carl-jung.net/alchemy.html. Accessed 17 August 2015.

Jung, C.J., von Franz, M.-L., Henderson, Joseph L., Jaffe, A. and Jacobi, J. (1964). *Man and His Symbols*. New York: Doubleday.

Khan, P.H. and Hasbach, P.H. (eds) (2012). *Ecopsychology: Science, Totems, and the Technological Species*. Cambridge, MA: MIT Press.

Kirschenbaum, H. and Henderson, V.L. (eds) (1990). *The Carl Rogers Reader. Reflections from the Lifetime Work of America's Preeminent Psychologist*. London: Constable.

LePera, N. (2021). *How to Do the Work: Recognise Your Patterns, Heal from the Past and Create Your Self*. London: Orion Spring.

Malchiodi, C.A. (2007). *The Art Therapy Sourcebook*. New York: McGraw-Hill.

May, R. (1994). *The Courage to Create*. London and New York: W.W. Norton and Company Incorporated.

McCarthy, D. (2012). *A Manual of Dynamic Play Therapy: Helping Things Fall Apart, the Paradox of Play*. London: Jessica Kingsley Publishers.

Mellon, N. (2000). *Storytelling with Children*. Stroud: Hawthorn Press.

Miller, A. (1990). *The Drama of Being a Child*. London: Virago.

Mills, J.C. and Crowley, R. (1986). *Therapeutic Metaphors for Children and the Child Within*. London: Brunner-Routledge.

Murray Parkes, C. (2008). *Love and Loss: The Roots of Grief and Its Complications*. London: Routledge.

Murdock. M. (1990). *The Heroine's Journey. Woman's Quest for Wholeness*. Boston: Shambhala.

National Association for the Education of Young Children (NAEYC) (2001). 'A conversation with Vivian Gussin Paley' (Online). Available at: www.naeyc.org/content/conversation-vivian-gussi((n-paley. Accessed 27 July 2015.

Pearson, C.S. (1991). *Awakening the Heroes Within*. New York: HarperCollins.

Piaget, J. (1999). *Play, Dreams, and Imitation in Childhood*. Hassell Street Press.

Play Therapy UK and Play Therapy International (PTUK and PTI) (2007). *Play for Life: The Journal of Play Therapy International and Its Affiliates*. Uckfield, East Sussex: PTUK.

Rae, T. (2020). *A Toolbox of Wellbeing: Helpful Strategies & Activities for Children, Teens, Their Carers & Teachers*. Banbury: Hinton House Publishers.

Rosen, M. (1993). *We're Going on a Bear Hunt*. London: Walker Books.

Salmon, P. (1995). *Psychology in the Classroom*. London: Cassell.

Sauder School of Business (2013). 'Want consensus in the boardroom? Get round a table' (Online). Available at: www.sauder.ubc.ca/News/2013. Accessed 27 July 2015.

Schaverien, J. (1991). *The Revealing Image: Analytical Art Psychotherapy in Theory and Practice*. London: Routledge.

Seyderhelm, A. (2020). *Helping Children Cope with Loss and Change: A Guide for Professionals and Parents*. Oxford: Routledge.

Shacham, M. and Lahad, O.A.M. (2012). *The 'BASIC Ph' Model of Coping and Resilience: Theory, Research and Cross-Cultural Application*. London: Jessica Kingsley Publishers.

Souter-Anderson, L. (2010). *Touching Clay, Touching What? The Use of Clay in Therapy*. Dorset: Archive Publishing.

Sunderland, M. (1999). *A Pea Called Mildred: A Story to Help Children Pursue Their Hopes and Dreams*. Oxford: Speechmark Publishing.

Sunderland, M. (2003). *Using Story Telling as a Therapeutic Tool with Children*. Oxford: Speechmark Publishing.

Taylor, B. (2003). *Forging the Future Together: Human Relations in the 21st Century*. Yorkshire: Oasis Press.

Therapeutic Puppetry. (2005). 'Therapeutic puppetry – empowering, transforming, healing' (Online). Available at: www.therapeuticpuppetry.com. Accessed 28 July 2015.

Tressider, J. (2003). *10001 Symbols. The Illustrated Key to the World of Symbols*, London: Duncan Baird Publishers.

Turner, B.A. (2005). *The Handbook of Sandplay Therapy*. Cloverdale, CA: Temenos Press.

Vogler, C. (2020). *The Writer's Journey: Mythic Structure*. Studio City, CA: Michael Wiese Productions.

Waters, T. (2004). *Therapeutic Storywriting: A Practical Guide to Developing Emotional Literacy in Primary Schools*. Abingdon: Routledge.

Wax, R. (2021). *A Mindfulness Guide for Survival*. London, Welbeck.

Whitfield, C.L. (1993). *Boundaries and Relationships: Knowing, Protecting, and Enjoying the Self*. Florida: Health Communications Inc.

Wikipedia (2012). 'House-Tree-Person Test' (Online). Available at: https://en.wikipedia.org/wiki/House-Tree-Person_test. Accessed 17 August 2015.

Winnicott, D. (1960). *The Maturational Processes and the Facilitating Environment*. London: Hogarth Press.

Wipfler, P. and Schore, T. (2016). *Listen: Five Simple Tools to Meet Your Everyday Parenting Challenges*. Palo Alto, CA: Hand in Hand Parenting.

Yasenik, L. (2012). *Play Therapy Dimensions Model: A Decision-Making Guide for Integrative Play Therapists*. London: Jessica Kingsley Publishers.

Young Minds (2020). 'Coronavirus: impact on young people with mental health needs. Survey 3: Autumn 2020 – Return to school'. Young Minds. Available at: https://www.youngminds.org.uk/media/0h1pizqs/youngminds-coronavirus-report-autumn-2020.pdf.

Index

Page numbers in italics refer to figures.